NATURAL BEAUTY

from the Outside In

SOJOURNER WALKER WILLIAMS

**STACKPOLE
BOOKS**

Guilford, Connecticut

STACKPOLE BOOKS

An imprint of Globe Pequot, the trade division of The Rowman & Littlefield Publishing Group, Inc.
4501 Forbes Blvd., Ste. 200
Lanham, MD 20706
www.rowman.com

Distributed by NATIONAL BOOK NETWORK
800-462-6420

British Library Cataloguing in Publication Information available

Library of Congress Cataloging-in-Publication Data

Names: Williams, Sojourner Walker, 1979– author.
Title: Natural beauty from the outside in / Sojourner Walker Williams.
Description: First edition. | Lanham, MD : Rowman & Littlefield Publishing
  Group, [2021] | Includes index. | Summary: "Many of the bath and beauty
  products we use contain toxic chemical substances, but it is easy to
  make your own safe, natural alternatives. In this book, Sojourner Walker
  Williams shares 75 of her most popular recipes"— Provided by publisher.
Identifiers: LCCN 2021010694 (print) | LCCN 2021010695 (ebook) | ISBN
  9780811739849 (paperback) | ISBN 9780811769785 (epub)
Subjects: LCSH: Beauty, Personal. | Herbal cosmetics. | Herbs—Therapeutic
  use. | Formulas, recipes, etc.
Classification: LCC RA776.98 .W55 2021 (print) | LCC RA776.98 (ebook) |
  DDC 646.7/2—dc23
LC record available at https://lccn.loc.gov/2021010694
LC ebook record available at https://lccn.loc.gov/2021010695

♾™ The paper used in this publication meets the minimum requirements of American National
Standard for Information Sciences—Permanence of Paper for Printed Library Materials, ANSI/
NISO Z39.48-1992.

First Edition

To my parents, Joanne and John, who named me
Sojourner and surrendered as I sprouted wings.

To Ohm, Jai, and Mark, who patiently shared
me with the pages of this book and joined in
adventures of testing recipes and picking herbs.

To N'Djamena and Mary, for their eyes,
insight, and guidance.

To all of my teachers and travel companions,
past and present, who have made this
lifetime a beautiful continuum of curiosity,
awareness, and adventure.

Thank you.

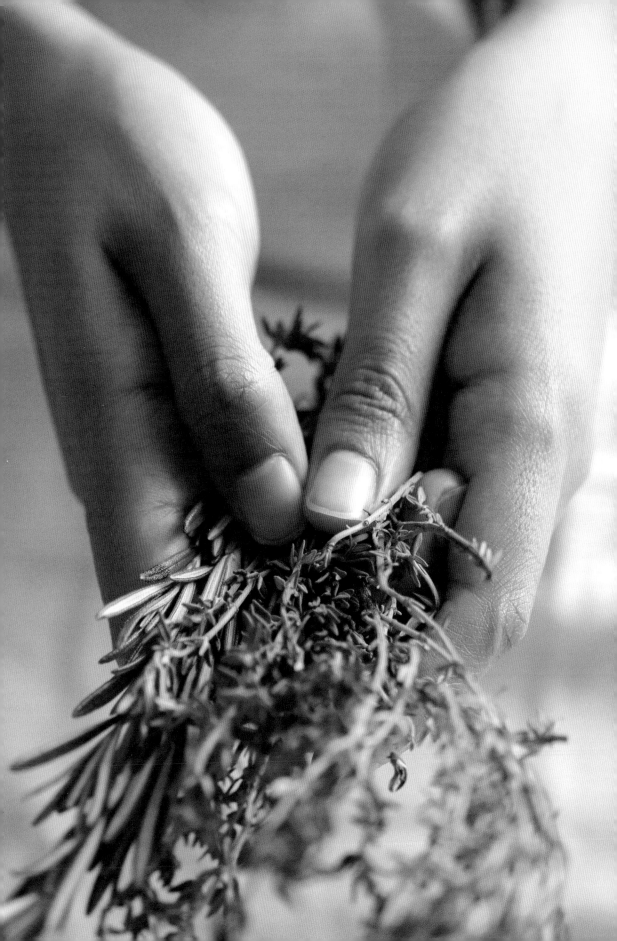

CONTENTS

Shea Butter / Ghana — 6

Coconut Oil / Thailand — 28

Herbs and Spices / Zanzibar — 39

Carrier Oils / Jamaica — 51

Floral Waters / Portugal — 66

Clay / Swaziland and France — 83

Essential Oils / New York City — 98

Aloe Vera / Costa Rica — 132

Vinegar Extractions / Japan — 144

Plant Barks / Mozambique — 151

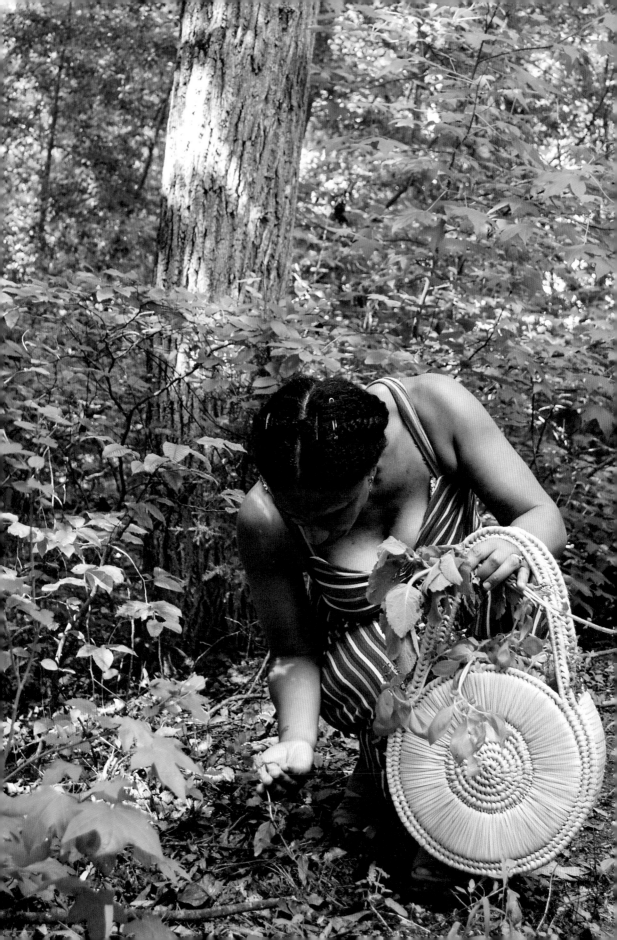

My toes sink into the rocky soil. The earth—firm, cool, and supportive—eases into the webbing between my toes. I can't resist the invitation for my body to soften and relax. I pause, let out a sigh, and gaze skyward. The air, misty and gray, clings to the space around me. The clouds overhead seal in the day's coolness, making it unusually pleasant for a late afternoon in August in the wetlands of southern Maryland.

The earth beneath my feet, so soft and receptive, is temporarily paralyzing. I almost don't want to move. It's my favorite time to be barefoot: after the rain. As I turn my palms to the sky, a light drizzle settles like dew on my skin. The sun, poising itself to break the tension cast from the recent thunderstorm, provides me with a small window of time to search for something that never seems to be where I last remembered it.

There is a rocky hill toward the western boundary of my property that's home to a wild blackberry bush. The bush is small and wide, sitting at the top of the hill near the back fence. I can visualize it but never remember its exact location. The landscape is constantly changing. I'd inherited the property wild and defiant, free of landscaping, and that's how it has stayed.

In most seasons, the birds and squirrels get to the blackberries before I can. Out of sight, there's a small and temperamental window for harvesting them. It's a time-sensitive mission.

"Two ounces," I whisper to myself—all I need to get the right shade is about two ounces of mashed ripe blackberries. But I have to move fast.

Back at the house, in the kitchen where I create, I've already melted my beeswax and shea butter for tinted lip balm sticks. In another 30 minutes, I'll be too late. And without the blackberries, I'll have to settle for no tint. I've run out of the pomegranate juice I used for the last batch, and I've been saving my beetroot powder for a jar of blush powder I'd promised to make for a friend.

The slope is steep, and my calves contract from the effort of the slippery

Taking a closer look at some basil.

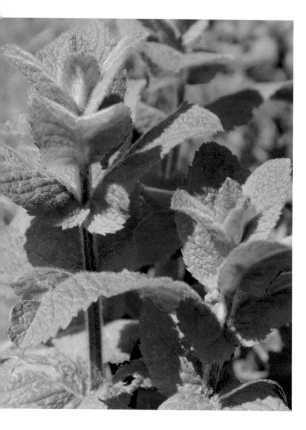

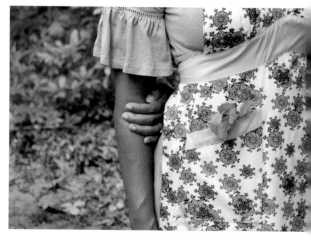

Foraging for peppermint.

At left: Peppermint.

barefoot climb. The landscape is ever changing this time of year, and I'm distracted by something out of place. A large black oak tree has fallen on its side, revealing a massive tangle of gnarled moss-covered roots. It's a piece of art. An entire world has come to life at the base of the tree. The poor thing must have fallen over a while ago, perhaps in the last storm, the wet earth easily churning over tree roots.

I freeze, heart slapping against my ribs at the sudden sensation of something crawling on my ankle. I imagine the culprit to be a large wolf spider, hairy and brown, the size of my hand, clutching my ankle bone with its eight monstrous, muscular legs. I jump back, hand lifted, adrenaline pumping, ready to strike. Instead, I burst into relieved laughter. It's only a vine of mint. Distracted by the fallen tree that barely missed the wood shed, I've

wandered right into my overgrown and poorly sectioned-off mint patch.

Mint is one of my favorite herbs. I find there's really no use trying to control its sturdy, sinewy vines. Why would you want to? Let it multiply. It was my trusted ground cover that blanketed my backyard slope in fragrant greenery. It spilled over the sides of pots placed around the deck and patio. There are hundreds of uses for mint. It always comes in handy. It smells amazing and is natural spider control. And then an idea comes. Reaching down, I separate three large fuzzy leaves from the stalk that has wrapped itself around my ankle—a pineapple mint variety. Pinching the base from where the leaves had been taken, I whisper, "Thank you," the sweet peppermint aroma stimulating my nostrils.

I place the leaves inside the mason jar in my apron pocket and continue the journey up the slope. Dragonflies circle a young magenta crepe myrtle tree. White hydrangeas, plump and shiny, weigh down the branches of the bush, whose thin, brown arms bend and buckle toward the ground in an effort to support their plump, blossoming weight. Past the path of yellowing creeping jenny, I spot a low tangle of vines clustered around the base of a silvery old cedar tree. Right away, I spy my prize. A shiny blackberry sits untouched, glistening with dew at the base of the prickly bush. But where are the others? Either I am late or the birds and squirrels have beaten me to the harvest. I crouch down and activate the flashlight on my iPhone to take inventory. There are only about five blackberries left to collect, and they are all deep inside the tangle of thorny brambles. Trying hard to control my imagination and block any images of wolf spider dens, I slide my hand inside the maze. Working carefully so as not to damage the fruit or cut my hands, I gather what I can. I manage to collect six berries. Not too shabby. They won't give me the dark tint I'm looking for, but they will do. I unscrew the lid, and the berries join the mint in the mason jar.

Fingers stained from collecting the overripe berries, I make my way back to the house, taking the rocky path that leads to my kitchen door. I've entered my sanctuary.

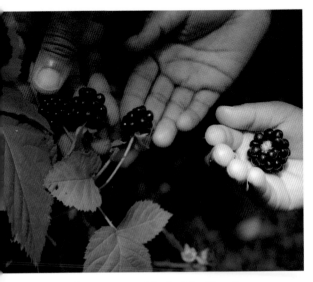

Careful not to squish the blackberries.

In my kitchen workshop, the sweet resin-like smell of beeswax hovers. I take a deep, appreciative breath. It's the aroma of creation. At the sink, I pull out a mini sieve and rinse the small and slightly shriveled blackberries and the hearty, fuzzy mint. Then I transfer them to my mortar and pestle; add a pinch of cinnamon, saffron, and turmeric; and begin to grind away.

The aroma, reminiscent of a rugelach pastry, is so enticing. The colors blend together harmoniously, taking on a new form; before long, I have a smooth, minty, wine-colored paste. Simmering on low in the double boiler, my shea butter and beeswax concoction is still warm. I add the freshly blended blackberry/mint paste to the pot, watching the crimson ripples that pulse around the blade of my hand mixer. The swirl of color and scent is glorious as the batter turns a pale wine hue. I pour the mixture into bamboo cases and seal them before placing them in the refrigerator to set.

A satisfied smile creases my lips. I make a cup of tea as I savor the magic of transformation—alchemy at its finest.

One day a week (more if it's holiday season, or if I have a large order to fill) for the last 13 years, I dedicate a few hours to hand making batches of natural skin care products. Similar to weekly meal prep, it's a ritual that began with my eye-opening introduction to Ayurveda.

⌐◞

On a Saturday afternoon 14 years ago, I was seated in class. I always chose the row on the far-right-hand side, the one closest to the window, three seats back, between my classmates Monica and Ashleigh. The classroom, a large gray square, was perched at the top floor of a creaky prewar building on University Avenue overlooking Union Square. Inside our classroom, the magic of transformation was unfolding. Ayurveda had cast a spell on me. The holistic Ayurvedic nutrition consultant training that I was taking was drawing me deeper and deeper into the mysteries of the natural world. Unraveling the science behind achieving balance was a fascinating and empowering journey.

Seven months into my yearlong training, my life was changing. I can't remember what exactly drove me to take the training. I'm not sure I truly even understood what Ayurveda was when I registered. An eighth-grade middle school teacher in the New York City public school system at the time, I suppose I was searching for my sanity.

I'd always been a yoga enthusiast. The philosophy of yoga—which I was just coming to explore—was interesting to me, and, naturally, Ayurveda (yoga's sister science, rooted in that same philosophy) engaged me both intellectually and spiritually.

The idea that all one had to do was look to nature to find the answers was deeply affirming. Learning to balance the elements around and inside us to both prevent disease and calm the mind was intriguing. According to Ayurveda, every living thing contains a life force energy and a constitution determined by the unique ratio of elements present in its makeup. Ayurveda recognizes the elements of water, earth, fire, air, and ether, and it is believed that at inception, a person, animal, or plant arrives in the world with a unique ratio of the elements, referred to as a constitution. This constitution (or *dosha*) dictates one's relationship to the world. For example, a person who has a lot of fire and air in their constitution

needs to eat foods and use body products that are cooling and grounding to balance out all of the heat and untethered air. Balancing elemental qualities effectively leads to mind, body, and spirit balance. So given that mint is cooling and cinnamon warming, a person with a lot of fire in their constitution would benefit from using cinnamon spice and cinnamon essential oil in moderation, as it only fuels their fire rather than pacifying and balancing it as mint would potentially do.

I found this new awareness infinitely fascinating. Ayurveda was exciting. A fatigued middle school English teacher, I was all about the pursuit of balance, which was at the heart of Ayurveda. Whether I was trying to understand the *doshas* (our unique elemental and energetic constitution blueprints—that is, how much air, earth, fire, water, and ether were present in our system) and *koshas* (the five layers of our subtle bodies—that is, the energetic and ethereal body, the "us" we can't see), or the different properties of foods, spices, seasons, and oils, there were so many lovely and intriguing nuances to dissect and try to understand. There seemed to be an infinite number of paths one could follow, and I was open to following each twist and turn until I found my footing.

This particular Saturday, after months of studying and identifying *doshas*/constitutions, *pranayama*/breathwork, meditation, cooking, and the prevention and treatment of disease with food, we were introduced to a unit on herbalism. With a background as an aesthetician, our instructor, Dr. Naina, expertly guided us on an herbal journey into the world of natural beauty, where we deconstructed recipe after recipe for handmade beauty products, salves, and tinctures.

Entranced, I watched Dr. Naina blend waxes and oils and infuse herbs and spices into ghee. A light went on as I came to the realization that this could be my niche. The heart of my Ayurvedic practice could lie in creating herb- and spice-infused natural beauty products. What a door to step through. It was 2007, and there was such a great need for educating people about the products they put on their skin. Nourishing ourselves from the inside out was much more intuitive than understanding how to nourish from the outside in. Creating products that drew from the earth's elements and abundance to promote natural beauty, purity, and balance was the greatest gift. It was in that classroom that the seeds for this book were planted.

At the end of my yearlong Ayurveda course, I became transformed into a handmade lotion–, face mask–, and facial/hair oil–making machine. I began concocting batches for myself. With my understanding of my *kapha/pitta* or earth/water/fire elemental constitution, I focused on patiently and lovingly addressing my skin's unique needs.

When I created a formulation I was satisfied with, I recorded every detail of the recipe and worked on developing new ones. I branched out into shampoos and conditioners, hand lotions, acne spot treatments, lip tints, and under-eye creams. In time, as my repertoire expanded, I began creating custom products for family and friends and eventually clients as well.

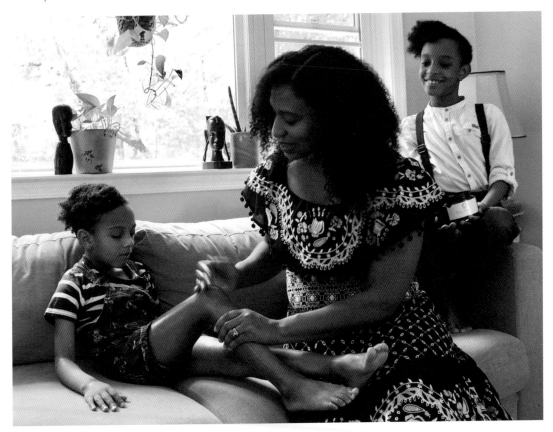

Soothing my son's eczema flare-up with a homemade cream.

Change is the only constant.

—Heraclitus of Ephesus

Ayurveda was a wonderful lens from which to first discover herbalism and natural skin and hair product formulations, but there was another influence at play that helped guide my journey as a maker of handmade bath and beauty products. Ayurveda opened my eyes, but it was my love for travel that fueled my creativity and curiosity. I began traveling right after college. Travel became my companion during that time of change, personal growth, and evolution. In many ways, the experience of traveling is like a mirror reflection of Heraclitus's famous quote, my then mantra—*change is the only constant.*

To travel is to embrace the present moment. Travel invites us to sink into and step outside of ourselves, engaging, as if for the first time, with new sounds, tastes, smells, sights, and textures. It's sensual and arousing; it's intellectually stimulating and humbling; and it's nurturing and grounding. Travel is evolution. It's balance.

I quickly learned that there were many different ways to travel. In addition to vacations and visiting friends, there was studying or living abroad. I had many stints during my early twenties, working as a traveling international educator. My Ayurvedic studies reignited my passion for travel, which in turn reaffirmed my desire to heal naturally.

Every new location had a mystery to reveal. That is what I love so much about travel. That, and perhaps the fact that my name is Sojourner, which literally means "one who sojourns," as in a person who travels from place to place, staying for a brief moment before moving on. In my case, this brief moment was at times six months, a year, a few short weeks, or a month.

My journey as a healer began in my mid-twenties and was a direct result of my travels. I developed a growing curiosity

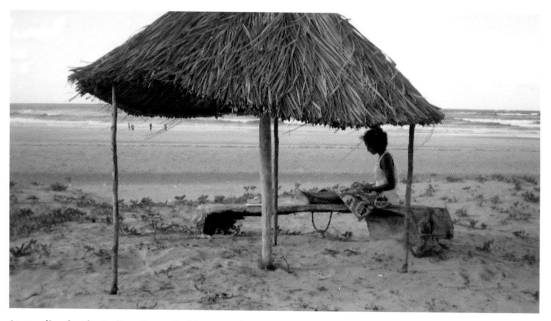

Journaling by the Indian Ocean in Morrungulo, Mozambique.

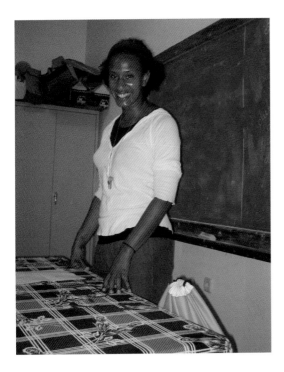

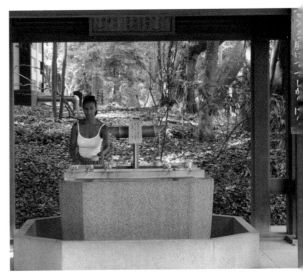

Osaka, Japan.

At left: Getting ready to teach my evening class in Inhambane, Mozambique.

about the many forms of natural, indigenous, and alternative herbal, spiritual, and medicinal practices I either witnessed firsthand or heard about through others. There were tales of medicine men in Ghana restoring a person's eyesight with plants. I watched in awe as a family in England treated a cold with herbs and homemade tinctures and teas just as the matriarch of the family three generations prior had taught them to do. I observed a mother in Barbados treat a child's digestive troubles with castor oil and roots. These interactions opened me up to a world of empowered possibility.

I moved beyond bath and body creations and began to dabble with herbs, reading books and taking workshops and courses in herbology. I was drawn to essential oils and took aromatherapy workshops and courses. I became a Reiki master. I embarked on the incredible journey to become a yoga instructor. Before I knew it, I was teaching yoga, healing with

Reiki, reading the Akashic records, giving Thai massages, deepening my intuitive understanding, and making herbal remedies, lotions, and body care products for family, friends, and clients.

I became the go-to woman in my circle when someone had a question about naturally treating an ailment and, later, when I became a mother, when someone had a question about naturally treating their child's minor illnesses and discomforts.

My love for travel was insatiable, and I continued to wander. I learned about spices while traveling through Zanzibar, Swaziland, and Mozambique. I learned about shea butter in Ghana. I learned about coconut oil and discovered new-to-me, local floral essential oils in Thailand.

No longer a New York City public school teacher, my sojourns became my muse. I created, tested, and refined products—products I reformulated years later to address the needs of my children's hypersensitive skin, and products that

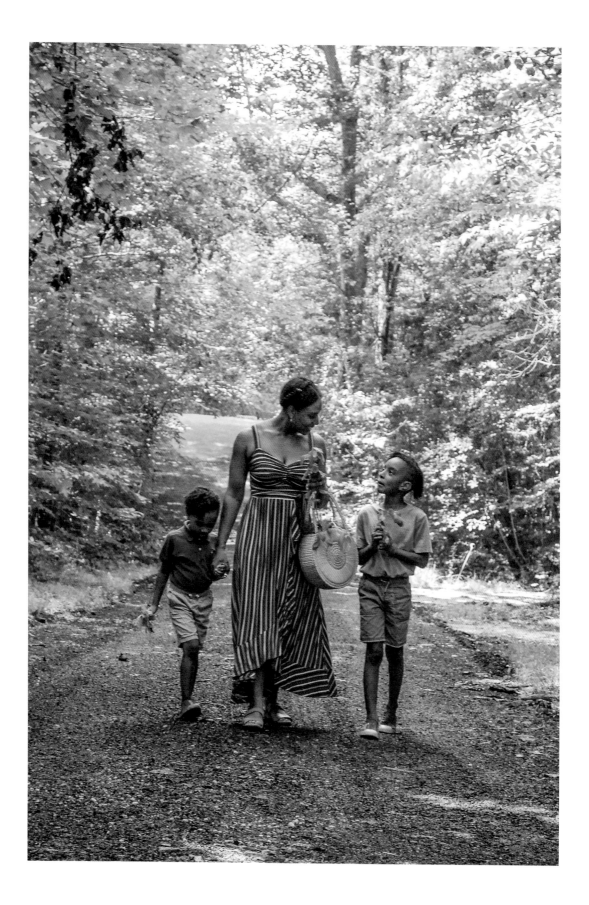

eventually, in 2009, turned into a natural body care line.

The joy and satisfaction that I've experienced in creating by hand the products that I choose to put on my body, just as a chef would prepare a meal, has been immense. Intentionally nourishing myself from the outside in, as well as from the inside out with the foods I ate, was so affirming. Knowing exactly what was in each of my daily products was a relief. Knowing that most of my body care was edible and that it was all nontoxic, and having the ability to create on-the-spot formulations to address my unique needs and the needs of my family with competence, confidence, and purity—whether dealing with eczema-prone skin, diaper rash, dandruff, acne, athlete's foot, or crow's feet—made me feel like an herbal superwoman.

This being said, and before you write me off as a recklessly militant DIYer, yes, I have a Western medical doctor, and yes, there are definitely times when I'm not able to take care of everything and I go to the doctor without hesitation. My degrees are in theater and education; I am not a medical doctor, and I don't claim to be. But for the small things, the minor afflictions, and as far as prevention is concerned, I step right in as women have done all over this great world for thousands of years. The results—better health for my family; soft, clear skin; shiny, thick hair; fewer colds and illnesses—speak for themselves.

We can all achieve this result. In these pages, I want to share some of what I've learned with you to show you how easy it really is to take charge of your health, create balance and vitality, and nurture beauty. This is everyone's birthright. This book was created for you, to be a resource guide, toolkit, and inspiration lab.

With clear, easy-to-follow recipes and research-backed explanations, *Natural Beauty from the Outside In* will hold your hand through every step of creating and adapting my recipes. These are all recipes you can create in your kitchen to nourish yourself and your loved ones from the outside in. We are, after all, not only what we eat but also what we put on our skin.

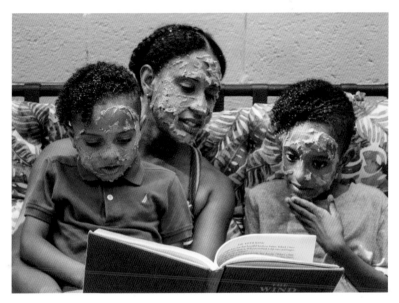

Cashew yogurt and green clay masks clump oddly but moisturize beautifully.

At left: Gathering herbs in the woods is a family affair.

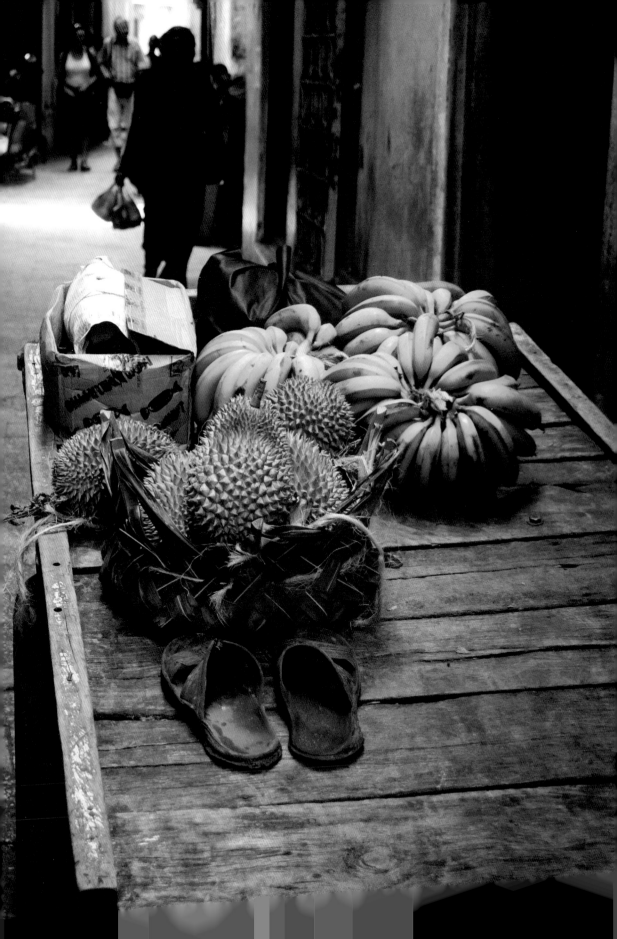

INTRODUCTION

*If we surrendered to earth's intelligence we
could rise up, rooted like trees.*

—Rainer Maria Rilke

Enormously strong and adaptable, yet surprisingly sensitive and easy to penetrate, your skin is your body's largest organ. An organ we can see and interact with. One that gives us direct and unmistakable feedback.

In the same way that we work carefully to nourish and care for organs like our heart and liver, equal care should be applied to our skin. When it comes to skin, most of us are connected on a cosmetic level. We focus on wrinkling and discoloration. We apply makeup and serums. It makes sense; we can directly see the results. But when it comes to feeding, cleansing, and detoxifying the skin externally, skin-purification uncertainty can arise. It's simply counterintuitive. All too often, we're taught to scrub and scrape at our skin, to slather it in paint and cover up everything perceived as an imperfection with a pretty, synthetic cosmetic Band-Aid.

Your skin is made up of three thick and hearty layers, and despite its ability to defend and protect, it is quite vulnerable. Our skin absorbs much of what is placed on the epidermis (outer layer), actively sucking anything it comes in contact with inside through the other two layers and into the bloodstream—hence the need for gloves when cleaning with commercial chemical agents. What if I were to tell you that some of the products you put on your skin and hair on a daily basis contain some of the same harsh chemicals?

While it's true that some chemicals are too large to penetrate through the three layers of skin, the vast majority of what is placed on your skin is small enough to be absorbed directly into your bloodstream and carried throughout your body. Your bath and beauty products may indeed be making you sick, but you have the ability to intervene and heal from the outside in.

When was the last time you read the ingredients on your shampoo, makeup, or lotion bottle? If you see in the ingredients list any of the following—parabens, phthalates, benzoyl peroxide, or triclosan, just to name a few common toxins—you will want to beware.

Parabens are preservatives commonly used in beauty formulations. Unfortunately, parabens are a hormone disrupter, known to interrupt estrogen production. In addition, parabens have been found in malignant tumors. Phthalates are also hormone disruptors. Typically listed as a fragrance, phthalates have been linked to reproductive difficulties and defects as well. Benzoyl peroxide is known to promote tumor growth and is an irritant to both skin and eyes, and triclosan is categorized by the Environmental Protection Agency as a pesticide—yuck. These and other hidden dangers can easily make their way into your bath and beauty products and can be causing damage to your health from the outside in.

I wrote *Natural Beauty from the Outside In* to present you with simple, clean, and natural alternatives to harsh, store-bought bath and body care products. Informed by my knowledge of Ayurveda, essential oils, and by my travels where I collected a treasury of traditional herbal healing techniques, I've curated my favorite and most effective recipes for you to try. In the same way that one plans a meal or prepares food for the week in large batches, you can address the nutritional needs of your hair and skin by making what you need for the week or month. Start small: pick one recipe that resonates, and commit to making that a part of your routine. When you're ready, add on until you have what you need.

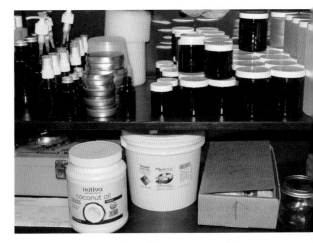

A peek into my bottle and jar storage cabinet.

Make space for creating and storing the ingredients you use. I keep a shelf and drawer in my kitchen for my DIY bath and body product supplies and ingredients. I use mostly mason jars and often recycle glass jars to store my creations.

Have fun, be creative, and add your own flair to these recipes. If the recipe calls for tea tree essential oil but you can't stand the smell of tea tree, don't use it. Use the basic recipe and add another essential oil you prefer. Oils, clays, and essential oils are chosen because of their properties and the way they complement the purpose of the product, but none of this has to be set in stone.

Any small step toward natural living is a good and courageous step. At the end of the day, it needs to feel right; own the process and your outcomes. Step bravely; step boldly. I'm here for you if you run into trouble.

HOW TO USE THIS BOOK

Natural Beauty from the Outside In is broken into chapters that feature a country and an ingredient endemic to it. Travelogue is used to introduce each region, inviting you, the reader, to experience both the country and the featured ingredient as I did when I first encountered it. In each section, I highlight how I have been impacted by the traditional healing wisdom of the area and how that experience influenced the products I make. You'll learn practical and detailed information about each featured ingredient, followed by easy-to-replicate recipes.

Resource guide, travelogue, and recipe book, *Natural Beauty from the Outside In* is yours to explore cover to cover, recipe to recipe, or section by section.

A PEEK INSIDE MY PANTRY

Before we get started with recipes, it might be helpful for you to peer into my pantry to get a sense of the tools and ingredients I use to make my bath and beauty products. I have a separate set of bowls, mixers, and supplies for my bath and beauty products, distinct from the ones I use for food preparation. In the beginning stages, this division is not necessary, but if you plan to take it to the next level and share or sell your products, you'll definitely want to ensure that there is no food contamination.

In the same spirit that one keeps certain staples in their kitchen, I keep the following tools and products stocked and ready to go for my weekly preparations.

TOOLS

- Multi-speed hand blender
- Wooden bowls and spoons
- Glass bowls
- Mortar and pestle (wooden or marble)
- Coffee grinder
- Glass measuring cups
- Ceramic measuring spoons
- Mason jars
- Amber and cobalt jars
- Sieve
- Cheesecloth
- Double boiler

PRODUCTS

- Shea butter
- Coconut oil
- Jojoba oil
- Sesame oil
- Almond oil
- Castor oil
- Calendula oil
- Black seed oil
- Sea buckthorn oil
- Essential oils (I have a large and revolving collection, but some of my staples are lavender, rose geranium, rose, jasmine, bergamot, lemongrass, frankincense, cardamom, sandalwood, peppermint, eucalyptus, spearmint, tea tree oil, chamomile, lemon, spikenard, vetiver, ylang-ylang, thyme, and oregano—you can pick your favorites)
- Carnauba wax and beeswax
- French green clay
- Bentonite clay
- Witch hazel
- Aloe vera gel
- Vitamin E
- Handmade floral waters, hydrosols, and tinctures (I have included my favorite recipes for you to experiment with)

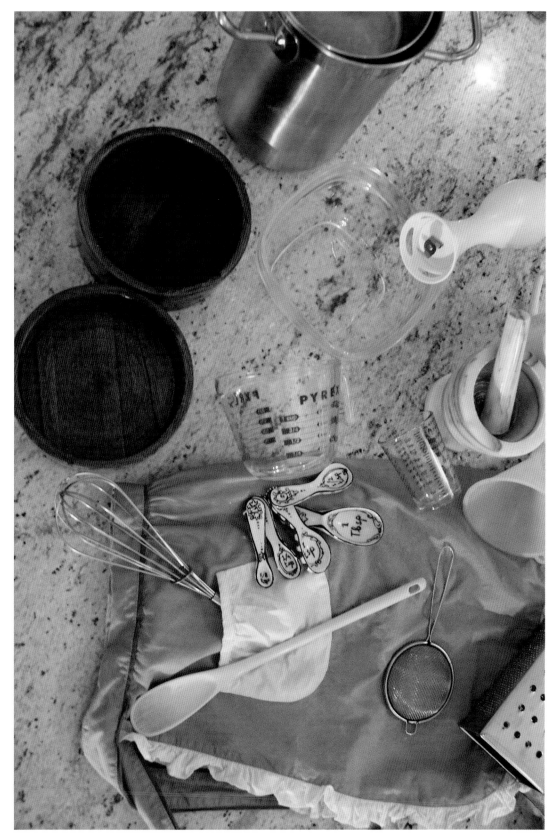

Here are some of the things you'll need to get started.

SHEA BUTTER
GHANA

West Africa, Summer 2005

"So-jah!"

I glanced up from my orange Fanta, wincing as the syrupy sweetness fizzed down my throat. I had just become used to the fact that my name, when spoken here, sounded like "soldier." Seeing no one in my immediate space, I continued to nurse my soda, which was disturbingly reminiscent of the pink antibiotic I used to take as a child every time I had an ear infection. It was hot. The humidity was heavy and suffocating. I wanted water but couldn't afford it. Tap water had the potential to make me violently ill. Bottled water was my only water option and was priced four times the already steep price of soda. That afternoon, I settled for soda. It didn't do the job.

Seated at the Cape Coast Café, I had a stunning view. I watched the waves of the Atlantic crash against the brown boulders that encircled the perimeter of the castle. Gray tufts of sea mist rose as a result of the spectacle. Ocean salt lingered on my lips. I purposely had left my book behind. I promised myself I would watch, listen, and take in this experience. It was my first time on the continent of Africa and my first attempt at traveling solo. Everything was new and exciting. Ghana was an awakening, and I vowed to accept, without distraction, the beauty around me.

"So-jah!"

I heard it again, closer this time. Turning my back to the Atlantic, I spotted a remotely familiar face in this new and still foreign space.

"Can I sit?" the man asked eagerly.

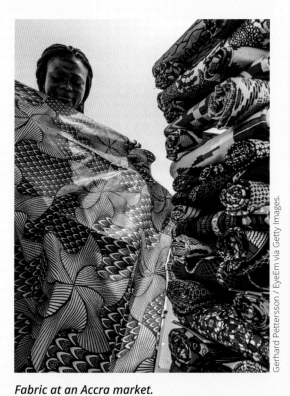

Fabric at an Accra market.

Gerhard Pettersson / EyeEm via Getty Images.

Woman at market stall.

Renate Wefers / EyeEm via Getty Images.

Shea butter being portioned for sale.

Godong/Stone via Getty Images.

I shifted nervously, trying to recall his name, place his features.

Despite my hesitation, and the fact that I had yet to reply, he made himself comfortable at my table.

"You look well, So-jah. Ghana is agreeing with you."

"Thank you." I smiled.

I felt as though Ghana was agreeing with me as well. I didn't know whether it was my new diet or the climate, but my skin had cleared and took on a new sheen, and I'd dropped about five pounds from all of the walking, literally upward of seven miles a day.

His eyes were playful and kind. I searched my head for his name. The details were filling in slowly. He was a drummer, a Rastafarian; we'd met once, maybe twice before, right here at the castle. He owned a shop with his brothers.

They sold drums and gave drumming and dance lessons mostly to British and French tourists. We'd talked a few weeks ago when I visited the castle to buy souvenirs after work with some of the other volunteers at the orphanage where I was teaching English. He had asked me where I was from, and he grew excited when I said New York. He had just been there; he had some cousins and a favorite uncle who lived in the Bronx. We had talked about being vegetarians. He'd lectured me about the virtues of cooking with coconut oil. How could I have forgotten? It had only been about two weeks ago. He, like most of the people I'd encountered in Ghana, remembered my name and looked me in the eyes with a warm smile while addressing me by name. Like many Americans, and like many Westerners, I let names roll in one ear and out the other and became embarrassed

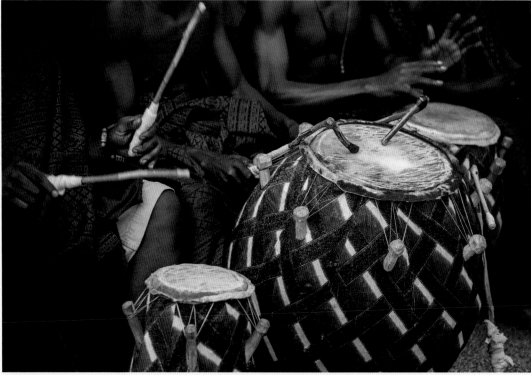

Ashanti drums in Kumasi, Ghana.

Anthony Pappone / Moment via Getty Images.

and apologetic when confronted by my instinctive and dismissive behavior.

"I'm so sorry," I finally managed. "What is your name again?"

His name was Eli. He lived in town. He was the youngest of seven children, five boys and two girls. His mother and grandmother owned the shop next to his. His father was from Burkina Faso.

We began to talk. Eli ordered a bottled water. I wanted water so badly. It was one of the great ironies I had learned to accept in Ghana. Fanta was cheap; almost everyone could afford it. Bottled water, because I couldn't drink from the tap, was fancy; it was overpriced and marketed to wealthy Westerners—not scrappy New York City public school teachers who spent their entire summer earnings on a plane ticket, having come to Ghana as a volunteer in dire need of conserving each penny.

I had another Fanta. The waves crashed. Flies buzzed. Skinny stray dogs settled at our feet.

"How is business?" I asked.

The long breaks in our conversation unnerved me.

"Business for me is very good." Eli smiled.

His teeth were pointy. He resembled a fox.

"So many English this time of year. They all want lessons. We have drumming and dance circles when the moon is full. You should come; they're here in front of the castle." He pointed with his water bottle to the open space before the castle.

"I'm not much of a dancer, but I'll come. I'd love to watch."

"You'll watch, but then you'll dance. You won't be able to stop yourself."

A hearty chuckle escaped my gut as I imagined myself gyrating and spastic,

dressed in *kente* cloth, backlit by the glow of the full moon. It wasn't a pretty vision.

"I want to show you something." Eli grew earnest.

"Yes?"

"Your face." He reached forward and touched my nose.

I recoiled, alarmed.

"I'm sorry. Did that hurt?"

The truth is it did hurt. But embarrassed by my reaction and not wanting to add to the awkwardness that I was feeling, I lied and said no.

Eli's face softened. "I was saying your face is too dry. Your skin is peeling."

I gaped at his blunt observation. It was all true, of course, but I hadn't expected him to point it out. I touched my nose. It was tender and inflamed.

"I'm peeling because I lost my sunscreen in Accra before I came here, and I haven't been able to find any more."

"Lost" was up for interpretation, since after arriving in the capital city, my sunscreen, shampoo, lotion, and a disposable camera were missing from my luggage.

"Sunscreen?" Eli's face wrinkled.

"You know, cream that protects your face and skin from the sun."

"That's what I want to show you." Eli was all smiles. "My mother's shop has the cream for your face."

"Your mother sells sunscreen?" I couldn't believe my luck. Sunscreen was so hard to come by.

"Shea butter." Eli announced proudly. "In Ghana, we use shea butter."

"Shea butter?"

I'd seen the curious white and yellow tubs at vendor stalls along 125th Street in Harlem, and I wasn't convinced. "I don't think I should put shea butter on my face."

"Of course. Why not?"

"It's too heavy. My skin will break out."

"You don't have to worry about that. Shea butter removes blemishes."

"But it's greasy."

"Not at all."

"No, it's definitely greasy." I frowned.

Eli laughed as if I'd just told a joke.

"Come, let's go to my mum's shop," he smiled.

Skeptically, I followed Eli's quick gait across the cobblestone road, through the gates of the Cape Coast Castle and into the shady courtyard that housed the artisan shops. I was led by hand into a small dimly lit nook. The three walls were lined with rickety shelves and stacked high with tubs of white, yellow, and brown.

An attractive, dark-skinned woman, whose age I couldn't gauge, popped out from behind a pile of cardboard boxes. She moved quickly, stepping forward and offering a greeting I didn't understand.

"Mama Sophia," Eli proudly announced, wrapping his arm around her shoulder.

I smiled. Mama Sophia wrapped me in a warm hug. She was simply stunning, surprisingly petite. I was drawn in by her bright eyes and shining skin. She couldn't have been more than five feet tall. Her eyes danced with childlike joy.

Eli exchanged slow words with his mother in Fante as she nodded and clicked her tongue in my direction.

"Sit." Sophia led me to a stool in the center of the room. She prepared a metal basin of water and, using a cloth, wiped at my face. I gripped the edge of my stool. Eli appeared cradling a marble-sized amber ball.

"This is black soap. It's good for your skin. You should use this. It works very well."

Before I had time to respond, Sophia was rubbing the black soap in enthusiastic

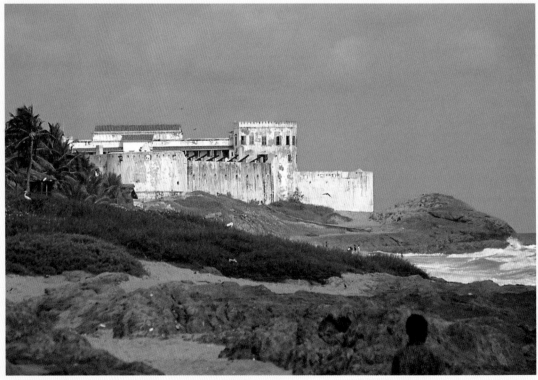

Cape Coast Castle, Ghana.

circles around my tender face. She rinsed the suds and then patted my skin dry with a towel.

"Feels good, doesn't it?" Eli was beaming.

It did feel good. My skin, heavy with humidity and sweat, was breathing. It felt alive and light.

"Close your eyes," Eli said, motioning to Sophia.

I did what I was told. Shea butter was massaged into my face under the direction of Sophia's firm hands. When she finished, I ran my fingertips across my forehead, swept them down my right cheek. My face wasn't greasy. My skin wasn't sticky or heavy; it didn't feel clogged.

Having nothing in particular that day to do, I watched for hours as Sophia, biceps bulging, packaged tubs of shea butter. Methodically, with a brisk flick of the wrist, Sophia used a wooden spatula to pry the compact butter from within a large dark gourd. Some of the shea butter gourds were yellow tinted, prepared with a turmeric mixture, while others were pure. Eli translated as I fired away with questions. I stayed until the shop closed and left that evening with a tub of shea butter and a tub of black soap.

Figuring I had nothing to lose, I set whatever facial cleanser I'd brought with me aside and began my black soap and shea butter regimen. Almost immediately, I stopped peeling and didn't burn as badly. Throughout the duration of my stay, I didn't experience a single nasty blemish, despite suffering from an onset of adult acne for months prior to my trip. Granted, my Ghanaian, non-processed food diet helped, but so did the shea butter. It provided a layer of nutrient-rich protection beneath the harsh Ghanaian sun.

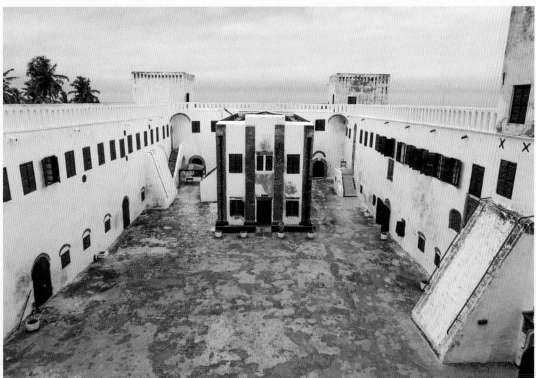

Elmina Castle, Ghana.

Merten Snijders / The Image Bank via Getty Images.

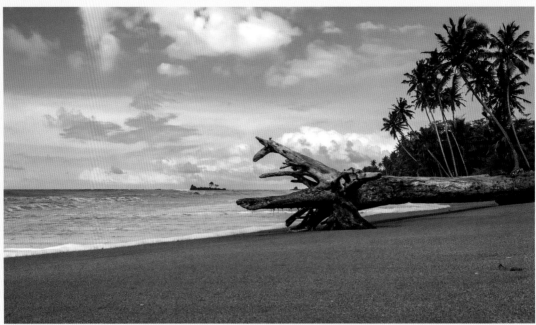

The Atlantic Ocean from the shores of the western coast of Ghana.

I visited Mama Sophia almost every day from that point forward. My serendipitous and unlikely introduction to shea butter marked the beginning of my shift toward all-natural and organic bath and body products. A few years later, when Dr. Naina revealed that she used shea butter in some of her Ayurvedic formulations, I thought back to Eli and Mama Sophia and smiled.

SHEA BUTTER 100% PURE AND UNREFINED

Thick, creamy, and slightly nutty in aroma, shea butter effortlessly glides over the surface of your skin, softening, lubricating, and creating a nourishing protective barrier. Like a batch of whipped goodness, pure shea butter melts into the skin without a trace, leaving a satin-like smoothness in its wake.

At more than 60% fat, shea butter is one of the most effective emollients, or skin softeners, out there. Its high fat content forms a rich and creamy consistency, and the emollient properties help it melt into and soften skin expertly.

At its essence, shea butter is a superfood derived from the seeds of the fruit that grow on the shea tree, which is endemic to West Africa. The seeds from the shea fruit are fertile with skin-loving vitamins like A, E, and F. Shea butter, resulting from the shea fruit seeds, is high in cinnamic acid, making it an effective anti-inflammatory agent useful in treating conditions from acne to arthritis. Full of essential fatty acids and the nutrients that support the production of collagen, shea butter is commonly used to reduce wrinkles and fight aging. Shea butter is high in oleic, stearic, palmitic, and linoleic acids that, with long-term use, are known to soften and smooth the skin. Deeply moisturizing, shea butter provides instant and long-lasting relief against dryness while protecting the skin's natural oils, even offering a low and naturally occurring dose of UV protection. Shea butter also is reported to have antitumor-promoting compounds called cinnamate esters, which, in addition to fighting inflammation, may be helpful in fighting tumors.

The shea tree is considered sacred by many tribes in Africa. The shea butter, an offering from the auspicious shea tree, has been used throughout centuries to protect skin from the harsh sun, wind, and dryness. Shea butter has also been used traditionally as a hair dressing, for wound care, to treat bug bites, and to treat leprosy. In addition, shea butter can be taken internally in the form of cooking oil or as a replacement for butter or lard in recipes.

Presently, both on and off the continent of Africa, shea butter is used to treat the following conditions:

- Eczema
- Dandruff
- Wrinkles and signs of aging
- Skin discoloration
- Acne
- Stretch marks
- Minor scrapes
- Bug bites
- Rashes

There are so many different ways to use shea butter in skin formulations. I'll share some of my favorite recipes in the following pages.

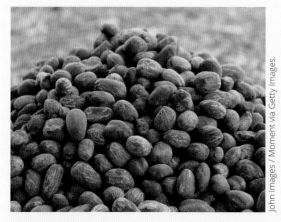

Shea butter seeds.

John Images / Moment via Getty Images.

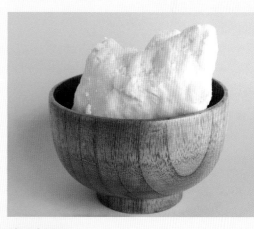

Shea butter.

Narcisa/E+ via Getty Images.

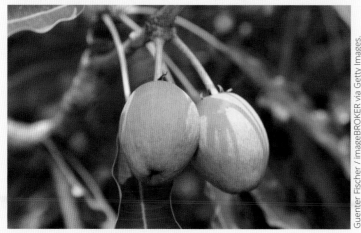

Guenter Fischer / imageBROKER via Getty Images.

Shea butter fruit.

SMOOTHING STICK DEODORANT

Moisturizing, calming, and fragrant, this is my go-to, first-thing-in-the-morning deodorant. It glides on easily and lasts the whole day.

WHAT YOU'LL NEED:

- 1 teaspoon beeswax (beads are easiest)
- 5 teaspoons shea butter
- 1 teaspoon vitamin E oil
- 2 teaspoons bentonite clay (don't use a metal spoon to scoop or mix!!!!)
- 1 teaspoon baking soda
- 15 drops lavender essential oil
- 10 drops cinnamon essential oil
- 5 drops frankincense essential oil

WHAT TO DO:

1. Melt the beeswax and shea butter together. The best way to do this is by using a double boiler. Place both the shea butter and beeswax in the boiler and heat on low until a liquid is formed.
2. Add vitamin E to the shea butter and beeswax liquid, and whisk until blended.
3. Add the bentonite clay and baking soda, and mix again using a non-metal whisk or spoon. Make sure to mix out any lumps; you want a thin consistency.
4. Next, add the essential oils to the mixture and mix once more.
5. Pour the liquid into an old, empty deodorant tube. I'm all about recycling, but if you haven't got a used tube, you can purchase them online.
6. Let the deodorant tube sit in the refrigerator for about an hour to set.

Yield:
One 1½-ounce deodorant tube

Preparation time:
90 minutes

Indications:
This is a gentle underarm deodorant. It is normal to experience perspiration, as this is not an antiperspirant formula.

Usage:
Apply to underarms in the morning or after showering.

Storage:
Store in a cool, dry place for up to a year.

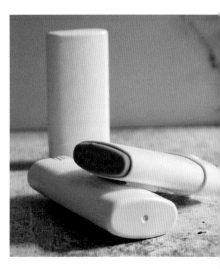

Smoothing Stick Deodorant.

SHEA BUTTER LOTION BARS

Thick and deeply moisturizing, lotion bars are great for winter skin and skin regularly exposed to the elements and irritants. Suitable for the most sensitive of skin, these lotions bars are for after-shower use and are designed to melt into warm skin.

WHAT YOU'LL NEED:

- ¼ cup shea butter
- ¼ cup olive oil
- ¼ cup beeswax
- Soap molds (any shape/variety you like)

WHAT TO DO:

1. Melt the shea butter, olive oil, and beeswax together in a double boiler on low heat.
2. Pour the mixture into soap molds and cool in the refrigerator for an hour.
3. Check to see that the bars are solid before taking them out of the refrigerator. You can wrap the bars in parchment paper and store in a cool, dry place until you're ready to use.

Yield:
Three 2-ounce bars of lotion

Preparation time:
90 minutes

Indications:
Lotion bars are great on warm, moist skin after a shower or on dry hands after washing dishes.

Usage:
Let lotion bar glide over skin, and then use your hand to rub in until absorbed.

Storage:
Store in a cool, dry place for up to a year. Avoid humidity and moisture.

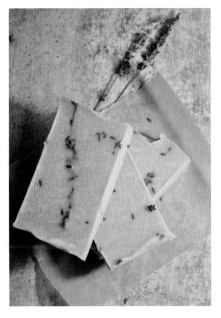

Shea Butter Lotion Bars.

MOISTURIZING SHAVING CREAM

Whipped and light, this moisturizing shaving cream will encourage a smooth shave and leave skin soft and silky afterward.

WHAT YOU'LL NEED:

- ⅓ cup shea butter
- ⅓ cup olive oil
- 2 tablespoons jojoba oil
- ¼ teaspoon vitamin E oil
- 10 drops lavender essential oil
- 1 tablespoon baking soda

WHAT TO DO:

1. Melt the shea butter and olive oil together in a double boiler. Add jojoba, vitamin E, and lavender essential oil.
2. Refrigerate (check in about 15 minutes and then every 5 minutes after that) until the mixture just begins to set.
3. Sprinkle baking soda over the top and blend with a hand blender.
4. Refrigerate a second time for 15 minutes. Blend again, using a hand blender, until whipped like frosting.

Yield:
6 ounces

Preparation time:
1 hour

Indications:
This thick shaving cream will help moisturize the skin and ensure a smooth shave.

Usage:
Apply a small amount to the desired area once it has been rinsed with water. Smooth a thin coating on before shaving.

Storage:
Store in a jar in a cool, dry place.

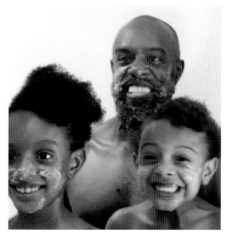

Moisturizing Shaving Cream: This cream is sensitive enough for the most aspirational of shavers!

BROWN SUGAR BODY SCRUB

A luxurious way to treat yourself in the shower, this gentle and exfoliating scrub sloughs away dead skin and softens skin. The floral, sweet aroma notes promote tranquility and ease.

WHAT YOU'LL NEED:

- ¼ cup shea butter
- ¼ cup jojoba oil
- ¾ cup brown sugar
- ½ teaspoon vitamin E
- 10 drops ylang ylang essential oil

WHAT TO DO:

1. Melt the shea butter in a double boiler over low heat.
2. Remove from the flame and add the jojoba oil, brown sugar, vitamin E, and ylang ylang essential oil.
3. Mix with a spoon.

Yield:
8 ounces

Preparation time:
20 minutes

Indications:
This is a gentle, soothing, and moisturizing body scrub.

Usage:
After showering, massage in a circular motion along the body. Rinse and follow up with your favorite lotion.

Storage:
Store in a cool, dry place for up to 6 months.

MOISTURIZING HAIR CREAM

Seal moisture into your hair shaft with this intensively hydrating and scalp clarifying cream. Ideal for curly, thick, and wavy hair types, this cream can be applied to damp hair before styling. A pea-sized amount can be applied to the scalp as well to increase blood flow, reduce dryness and itchiness, and promote hair growth.

WHAT YOU'LL NEED:

- ½ cup shea butter
- ½ cup castor oil
- ⅛ cup jojoba oil
- 10 drops lavender essential oil
- 10 drops peppermint essential oil

WHAT TO DO:

1. Melt the shea butter in a double boiler on low heat.
2. Remove from the flame and add castor oil, jojoba oil, and the lavender and peppermint essential oils.
3. Mix with a hand mixer until creamy.

Yield:
One 8-ounce jar

Preparation time:
15 minutes

Indications:
This smoothing and softening pomade seals in moisture and helps enhance any natural curl or wave pattern that may be present.

Usage:
Apply a small amount to your hair by rubbing it in your palms and smoothing over hair. Best used on damp hair.

Storage:
Store in a cool, dry place for up to a year.

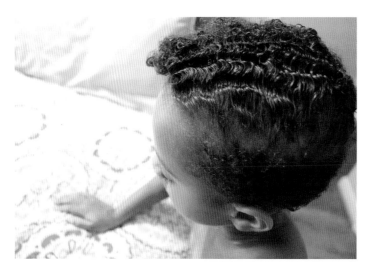

Moisturizing Hair Cream: This cream creates tangle-free tresses, even in curly and wavy hair.

CURL-DEFINING HAIR GEL

Give your curls definition and polish with this light and fragrant gel. Light enough for fine curl textures as well as thick, this gel is nondrying and provides a strong, sleek hold that will not flake. Note: This recipe pairs well with the Moisturizing Hair Cream (see page 18).

WHAT YOU'LL NEED:

- ¼ cup shea butter
- 2 tablespoons raw honey (diluted in a tablespoon of boiling water)
- ½ cup sweet almond oil
- 20 drops rosemary essential oil

WHAT TO DO:

1. Melt the shea butter in a double boiler over low heat, and then set aside.
2. Dilute the 2 tablespoons of raw honey into 1 tablespoon of boiling water.
3. Add the shea butter, sweet almond oil, and rosemary essential oil.
4. Pour into a bowl and mix thoroughly until smooth and uniform.
5. Refrigerate for 20 minutes until just about set, and then blend and whip with a hand blender.
6. Refrigerate again for 15 minutes, and then whip a second time with a hand blender before transferring to a storage container of your choice.

Yield:
6 ounces

Preparation time:
1 hour

Indications:
This whipped cream helps define and enhance your natural curl pattern. The honey provides a gel-like hold without being hard and crusty thanks to the shea butter and almond oil.

Usage:
Apply to wet hair from root to tip after conditioning.

Storage:
Store in a cool, dry place for up to 2 months.

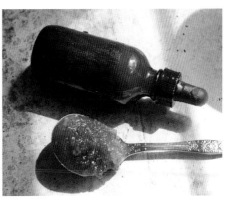

Curl-Defining Hair Gel.

STRETCH MARK CREAM

This concentrated cream is a double dose of prevention and treatment. Apply to stretch mark–prone skin daily to prevent new marks and gradually fade and reduce the appearance of old ones. This blend is gentle enough for pregnant bellies.

WHAT YOU'LL NEED:

- ¼ cup shea butter
- 2 tablespoons vitamin E oil
- 10 drops lavender essential oil
- 10 drops myrrh essential oil
- 10 drops frankincense essential oil

WHAT TO DO:

1. Melt the shea butter in a double boiler over low heat.
2. Add the vitamin E oil and essential oils.
3. Hand blend to a whipped consistency.
4. Transfer into a container.

Yield:
2½ ounces

Preparation time:
30 minutes

Indications:
This stretch mark cream can be used as a preventative as well as a treatment. The shea butter and vitamin E oil work to provide elasticity to the skin to help avoid the likelihood of stretch marks in stretch mark–prone areas. The frankincense and shea butter also help reduce the appearance of preexisting stretch marks due to their cellular-regenerating properties.

Usage:
Apply to stretch marks or areas prone to stretch marks twice daily (morning and evening).

Storage:
Store in a cool, dry place for up to a year.

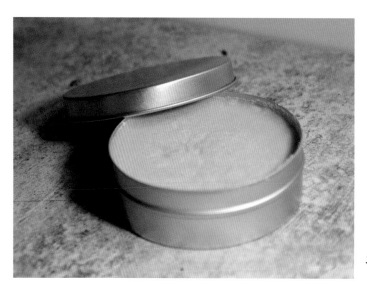

Stretch Mark Cream.

CUTICLE SOFTENER

Relieve dry, peeling cuticles with this restorative cream formula that will restore moisture and elasticity as well as provide antiseptic properties to heal hangnails and fissures.

WHAT YOU'LL NEED:

- 1 teaspoon shea butter
- 5 drops eucalyptus essential oil

WHAT TO DO:

1. Melt the shea butter in a double boiler (or Pyrex bowl placed inside a pot of boiling water).
2. Once a liquid has been formed, add 5 drops of the eucalyptus oil to the melted shea butter. Stir and pour into a ½-ounce metal tin.
3. You can cool and set your cuticle cream by placing it in the refrigerator for 20 minutes.

Yield:
½ ounce

Preparation time:
30 minutes

Indications:
This cream helps soften cuticles and reduce hangnails and peeling.

Usage:
Apply a small amount as needed to cuticles and massage until fully absorbed.

Storage:
Store in a cool, dry place for up to a year.

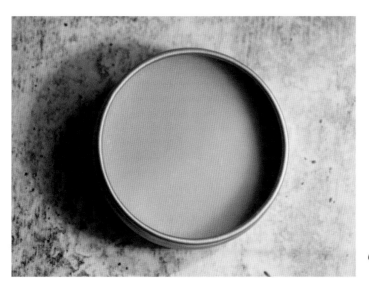

Cuticle Softener.

WHIPPED BODY BUTTER

This light, cooling, and creamy moisturizing lotion softens skin without leaving a greasy residue. This blend is particularly effective when used during the spring and summer months or in warmer climates.

WHAT YOU'LL NEED:

- 1 cup shea butter
- ½ cup unrefined coconut oil
- ½ cup almond oil
- 1 teaspoon vitamin E oil
- 15 drops of essential oils of choice

WHAT TO DO:

1. In a double boiler, melt the shea butter and coconut oil together. Once melted, cool at room temperature until the mixture begins to stiffen (20–30 minutes).
2. Stir in almond oil, vitamin E oil, and essential oils.
3. Cover and place in the freezer to set. You'll need to monitor the mixture as it sets. You're looking for the mixture to turn lighter and begin the process of solidification. Usually there's a ring around the periphery of the container of the stiffest lotion and a slight depression at the center, a bit darker and oilier. When this happens, remove from the freezer.
4. Whip with a hand blender until there's a fluffy, buttery texture.

Yield:
16 ounces

Preparation time:
90 minutes

Indications:
Whipped body butter is a light, creamy, and intensely moisturizing body treatment.

Usage:
Rub the desired amount over your body after a shower or whenever moisture is needed.

Storage:
Store in a cool, dry place for up to 6 months.

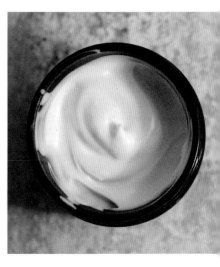

Whipped Body Butter: It's so silky!

BODY BUTTER

Rich and deeply moisturizing, this body butter recipe will leave skin soft and hydrated even in the driest of climates. This is an ideal late autumn and winter weather lotion.

WHAT YOU'LL NEED:

- 1 cup shea butter
- ½ cup unrefined coconut oil
- ¼ cup olive oil (or carrier oil of choice)*
- 1 teaspoon vitamin E oil
- 15 drops of essential oils of choice

*See page 58 for a list of carrier oils.

WHAT TO DO:

1. In a double boiler, melt the shea butter and unrefined coconut oil.
2. Allow the mixture to cool at room temperature until it begins to stiffen (20–30 minutes).
3. Add the olive oil, vitamin E oil, and essential oil.
4. Use a hand blender on low to blend.

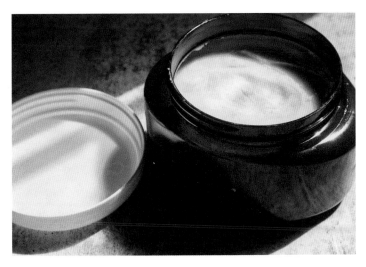

Yield:
16 ounces

Preparation time:
45 minutes

Indications:
This is the ultimate in body moisturizing. Thick, soothing, and creamy, this butter will moisturize without being greasy and will provide moisture all day long, even throughout the dry, cold winter months.

Usage:
Apply desired amount to your body after bathing or whenever moisture is needed. You may need to rub the butter in your palms to soften before application if the storage temperature is cold.

Storage:
Store in a cool, dry place for up to a year.

Body Butter.

FACIAL MOISTURIZER FOR MATURE SKIN

Designed to address the unique needs of mature skin, this facial moisturizer is gentle, hydrating, collagen stimulating, antioxidant rich, and calming.

WHAT YOU'LL NEED:

- 1 cup shea butter
- ½ cup sea buckthorn oil
- ¼ cup tamanu oil
- ¼ cup calendula oil
- 1 teaspoon vitamin E oil
- 10 drops frankincense essential oil
- 5 drops myrrh essential oil

WHAT TO DO:

1. In a double boiler, melt shea butter and set aside to cool for about 30 minutes.
2. Add sea buckthorn oil, tamanu oil, calendula oil, and vitamin E oil.
3. Add frankincense essential oil and myrrh essential oil.
4. Blend with a hand mixer on low until uniform.

Yield:
16 ounces

Preparation time:
45 minutes

Indications:
This blend helps maintain a smooth, youthful appearance. The unique blend of carrier and essential oils work together to spark cellular regeneration, improve circulation, soften, brighten, and reduce pores. The oils absorb quickly without leaving a greasy residue.

Usage:
Apply to face, neck, and the backs of hands once or twice daily.

Storage:
Store in a cool, dry place for up to a year.

NATURAL SUNSCREEN

This natural sunscreen formula is ideal for everyday moderate sun exposure and provides a natural SPF around 25. Suitable for use on both face and body, this sunscreen provides just enough protection for everyday limited sun exposure. Note: If you plan to be outdoors for an extended period of time, you will want to reapply every hour or so. If you will be exposed to intense sun or are in a heavy UV index area, you'll want to take further protective measures and cover exposed skin.

WHAT YOU'LL NEED:

- 1 ounce shea butter
- 2 ounces tamanu oil
- 1 ounce carrot seed oil

WHAT TO DO:

1. In a double boiler, melt the shea butter and set aside for 5 minutes to cool.
2. Add tamanu and carrot seed oil.

Yield:
4 ounces, glass pump bottle

Preparation time:
10 minutes

Indications:
Carrot seed oil has a natural SPF between 30 and 40, and tamanu oil has a natural SPF around 20. This oil blend works together to provide biological UV protection.

Usage:
Apply oil to exposed skin before going outside or before sun exposure. Reapply every hour for continuous protection during prolonged exposure. Avoid eyes and mouth.

Storage:
Store in a cool, dry place in a tinted glass bottle for up to 6 months.

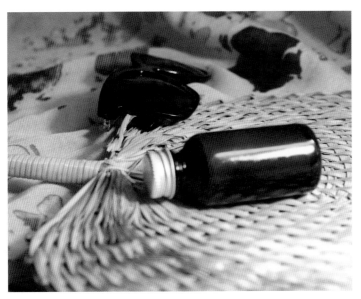

Natural Sunscreen: Fun in the sun without the bluish tint with this natural sunscreen.

BEARD-REFRESHING CREAM

Even beards need some love from time to time. This light, shine-enhancing, and detangling formulation will help soften and freshen even the wildest beards. With antimicrobial and antibacterial properties to keep germs away from the face, the beard-refreshing cream's aromatic woodsy scent is also grounding and calming. This formula also helps protect against ingrown hairs—BONUS!

WHAT YOU'LL NEED:

- ¼ cup shea butter
- 1 tablespoon jojoba oil
- ⅛ cup sweet almond oil
- 5 drops cedarwood essential oil
- 5 drops sandalwood essential oil
- 3 drops vetiver essential oil

WHAT TO DO:

1. In a double boiler or in a Pyrex glass container placed into a pan filled with about an inch of boiling water, melt the shea butter to a liquid.
2. Combine the liquid shea butter, the jojoba oil, the sweet almond oil, and the drops of essential oils into your container. Fasten the top and shake vigorously until well blended.
3. Refrigerate for 20 minutes until set, and then return to room temperature.

Yield:
3½ ounces

Preparation time:
30 minutes

Indications:
This cream naturally cleans, deodorizes, and conditions beard hair.

Usage:
Apply a small amount to beard before grooming. A pea-sized amount, rubbed on the palms and then smoothed over a beard, will make the skin beneath silky smooth and will condition and lightly scent even the grungiest of beards.

Storage:
Store in a cool, dry place for up to a year.

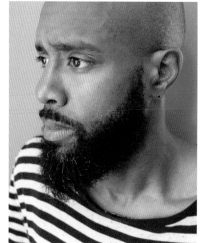

My partner's favorite product!

Far right: Beard-Refreshing Cream.

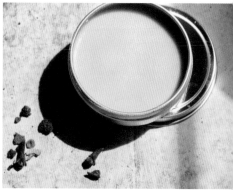

ANTI-AGING FACIAL CREAM

This soothing cream is designed to protect your skin from the signs of aging. This can be used at any age to support and maintain a healthy, youthful glow.

WHAT YOU'LL NEED:

- ½ cup shea butter
- ½ teaspoon sea buckthorn oil
- ⅛ teaspoon turmeric
- 35 drops of frankincense essential oil

WHAT TO DO:

1. Melt the shea butter in a double boiler over low heat or by using a Pyrex glass container placed inside a pot filled ¼ of the way with boiling water.
2. Once the shea butter has turned to a liquid, pour it into a container. Add the sea buckthorn oil, turmeric, and frankincense.
3. With the lid secured tightly, shake the mixture until the contents have blended thoroughly. It should be a light gold color.
4. Place the container in the refrigerator for 30 minutes to set before returning it to a room temperature environment.

Yield:
4 ounces

Preparation time:
45 minutes

Indications:
This cream helps fight the signs of aging, preserving the skin's youthful appearance while encouraging rapid cellular regeneration and moisturizing.

Usage:
Apply a small amount to face and neck once or twice daily.

Storage:
Store in a cool, dry place for up to a year.

COCONUT OIL
THAILAND

I wasn't always a beach person. For the first 20 years of my life, I liked the idea of the ocean and of the rolling waves, but I had never had a moment of true connection. The beaches near Lake Ontario, where I grew up, were ice cold and murky, and they smelled funny. The beaches in New York City, though a welcome break from the hectic pace of life, were crowded and noisy and just didn't soothe me.

Then I visited Thailand—the pristine island of Khao Lak, to be specific. It was as if I saw the water, the ocean, for the first time. The Andaman Sea, turquoise and lilting, was warm. The gentle waves, playful and inviting, called to me. Stepping into the sea, I could wade serenely chest deep. From my waist to my feet, I could see subtle, shimmering layers of water and life.

I first visited Thailand in 2006, a few short months after the terrible Asian tsunami. My friend Susan was doing development work in the region, and I was invited to pitch in. Even then, after all the destruction, like a rainbow at the end of a storm, Thailand was radiant.

I've made several trips to Thailand since then, and after each one, I'm compelled to return. A visceral place, there is so much to taste, smell, touch, hear, and see, and despite the distance, I am drawn back to this place of overwhelming beauty.

In Thailand, I was introduced to coconuts—really introduced, as in I'd spend about an hour walking, sitting, and striking a yoga pose or two through dense coconut groves on my way to the ocean. The sweet smell of coconut wafting in the breeze from fallen coconuts that split open upon landing on the ground, a pool of clear sweet milk creating canals through the black soil. Everywhere, there

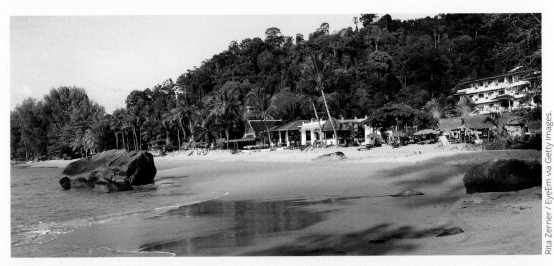

Beach on the Andaman Sea, Thailand.

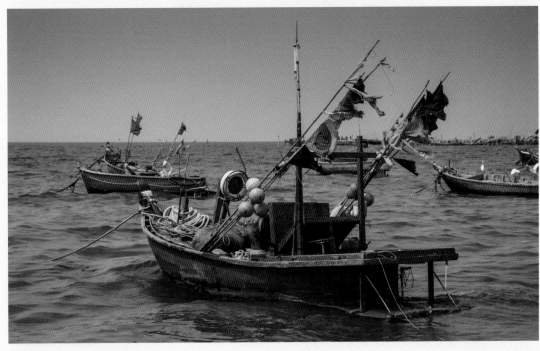

Fishing boats, Thailand.

seemed to be trees, heavy with coconuts. The air in the countryside of Khao Lak was perfumed by coconuts with a hint of jasmine and a splash of lemongrass.

I drank my first raw coconut in Thailand. How I had managed so long without experiencing sweet coconut water taken directly from a round coconut warm from the sun, I'll never know. The coconuts in Thailand yielded the sweetest, most energizing water. The warm liquid, like the milk of life, cooled me from the inside out. It didn't matter that it wasn't ice cold; there was something so placating about the life force of the coconut. It was everywhere—in beverages, in the air, in food. Coconut made even the most chili-infused curry soft and inviting. Coconut was like the moon—calm, cool, and maternal.

Thailand is a country steeped in a rich tradition of healing techniques. Thailand has its own form of traditional medicine uniquely influenced by Ayurveda and Chinese medical systems. Thai massage is a branch of Thailand's traditional medical practice. And it was here, on the beach, the Andaman Sea in the distance, that I would indulge in a full-body Thai massage almost every day.

It was an indescribable experience, with the roaring sea in the distance as I reclined upon a flat cushion swathed in colorful silk, lulled into a deep meditative bliss. During the massage, coconut oil was rubbed into my skin, while every care, every stress, was released into the

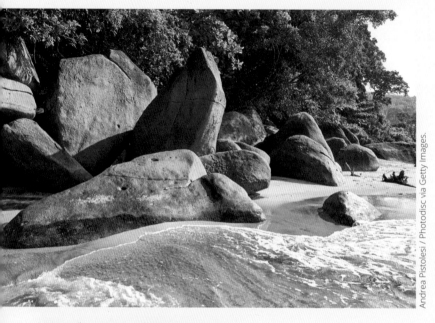

Andrea Pistolesi / Photodisc via Getty Images.

Beach at Khao Lak, Thailand.

Below: Asian elephants.

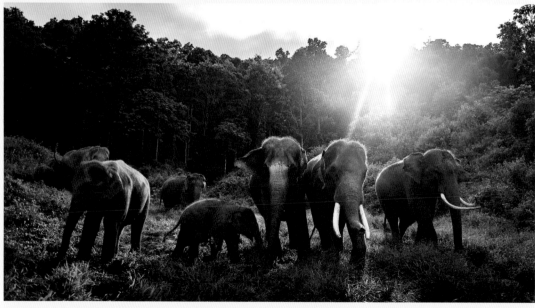

Skaman306 / Moment via Getty Images.

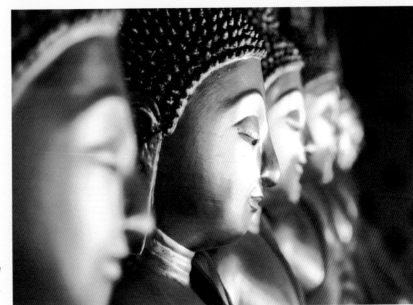

Buddhas in Bangkok, Thailand.

ether through acupressure, deep tissue massage, and full-body stretching and pulling. With energy healing at its finest, my jet lag subsided, my hot skin cooled and my soul soothed; these massages were 90 minutes of pure perfection. Daily massages were a luxury I couldn't dream of being able to afford in New York City, but at around US$15 a session, they were factored into my budget in Thailand.

When after a few days I ran out of my travel-sized lotion, instead of running to the 7-Eleven in town, which was stocked with Western products, I asked the woman who gave me my massages what lotion she used when she massaged my skin. It smelled wonderful and left my skin soft and hydrated. She pointed me in the direction of a local artisan coop shop where her sister sold a coconut lotion product. The shop, a fair trade collective of local artists, healers, and craftsmen affected by the tsunami, became the mecca where I first discovered the power of coconut oil.

Prior to my trip to Thailand, I rarely even cooked with coconut oil, and suddenly I was rubbing it on my skin and hair, drinking hot beverages with it, and eating food cooked in it. Coconut oil was a staple in most of the lotions and body care products at the shop. In Thailand and many other Southeast Asian countries, coconut oil is a cosmetic and medicinal go-to and takes on so many iterations: pure and unrefined (no processing or diluting), fractionated (liquid as a result of the long chain fatty acids being removed), or blended with essential oils or diffused with herbs.

During my many visits to the shop, I asked questions and bought products— lots of products. I bought lotions blended with jasmine and essential oil of frangipani. I bought oils blended with lemongrass, eucalyptus, and basil. I took notes on their intended uses, tested them on my skin, and blended them with my own handmade products. The experiments were thrilling. When I returned to New York, coconut oil became a part of my regular routine.

COCONUT OIL 100% PURE AND UNREFINED

Light, fragrant, and moisturizing, coconut oil has been a staple ingredient in skin care in Southeast Asia for centuries. Naturally antibacterial and antifungal, coconut oil has the ability to deeply detoxify and cleanse the skin, treating and preventing certain bacteria and fungi. Coconut oil penetrates both skin and hair effortlessly. When it comes to the most penetrating oils for the hair, coconut oil is one of the best at penetrating and moisturizing the hair shaft. Coconut oil is high in capric, caprylic, and lauric acids, which are fatty acids with powerful disinfectant and antimicrobial properties. These qualities explain why coconut oil is often a favored option when it comes to oil pulling (an Ayurvedic practice for oral hygiene and detoxification). Coconut oil is rich in vitamin E and packed with protein, which contributes to cellular health, tissue repair, and the restoration of damaged skin cells. It is a staple in Ayurvedic medicine.

Presently, in Southeast Asia and beyond, coconut oil is used to treat the following:

- Psoriasis
- Scarring
- Eczema
- Skin infections
- Bacterial and fungal infections
- Aging
- Hair frizz
- Dry hair
- Wounds

There are so many different ways to use coconut oil in skin formulations. I'll outline some of my favorite recipes in the following pages.

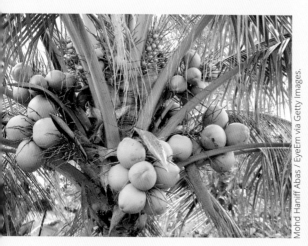

Coconuts on a palm tree.

At right: Palm tree grove.

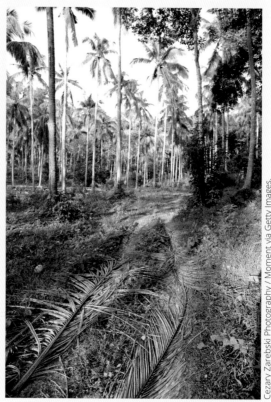

Mohd Haniff Abas / EyeEm via Getty Images.

Cezary Zarebski Photography / Moment via Getty Images.

WHIPPED COCONUT AND ALOE BODY LOTION

This is a very light and soothing lotion ideal for summertime use. The aloe assists in calming sun-sensitive skin, while the coconut oil cools. This is also an ideal lotion to apply after shaving the legs or face.

WHAT YOU'LL NEED:

- ¾ cup softened unrefined coconut oil
- ¼ cup aloe vera gel
- ½ teaspoon vitamin E oil
- 5 drops essential oil of choice

WHAT TO DO:

1. If your coconut oil is hard, soften it by running the jar under warm water.
2. With a spoon, mix the coconut oil, aloe vera gel, vitamin E, and essential oil until thoroughly blended.
3. Refrigerate for 10 minutes.
4. Whip by blending with a hand blender on high to a frosting-like consistency.

Yield:
8 ounces

Preparation time:
20 minutes

Indications:
This formulation is light, absorbs quickly into skin, and provides light to medium moisture.

Usage:
Apply after bathing or when needed.

Storage:
Store in a cool, dry place for up to 3 months.

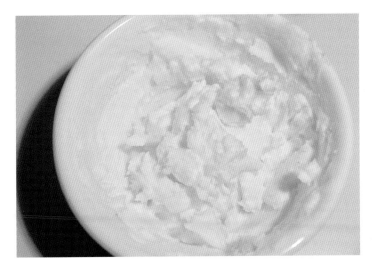

Whipped Coconut and Aloe Body Lotion: It's light and nongreasy.

WHIPPED BODY LOTION FOR MATURE SKIN

This moisturizing, antioxidant-rich, and skin-regenerating whipped body lotion recipe is designed to address the needs of mature skin.

WHAT YOU'LL NEED:

- 1 cup softened unrefined coconut oil
- 2 tablespoons vitamin E oil
- 20 drops frankincense essential oil

WHAT TO DO:

1. If your coconut oil is hard, soften it by running the jar under warm water.
2. In a bowl, combine coconut oil, vitamin E oil, and frankincense.
3. Place the mixture in the refrigerator for about 10 minutes.
4. Whip by using a hand blender to mix on high to a whipped consistency.

Yield:
8 ounces

Preparation time:
20 minutes

Indications:
This lotion is light, provides medium moisture, and encourages rapid cellular regeneration.

Usage:
Apply as needed or after bathing to face and body.

Storage:
Store in a cool, dry environment for up to 6 months. If your lotion begins to melt due to warm temperatures, place in the refrigerator for 5 minutes to set.

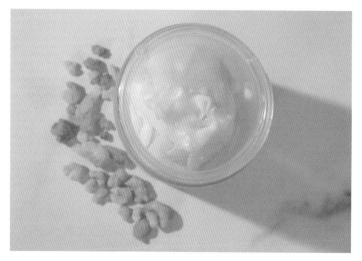

Whipped Body Lotion for Mature Skin.

TOOTHPASTE

Refreshing, whitening, and promoting remineralization, this toothpaste will condition gums and keep your mouth healthy.

WHAT YOU'LL NEED:

- 1 tablespoon bentonite clay
- 2 tablespoons baking soda
- 3 tablespoons unrefined coconut oil
- 10 drops peppermint essential oil

WHAT TO DO:

1. In a glass bowl, mix the bentonite clay and baking soda with a non-metal spoon (metal deactivates bentonite clay).
2. In another bowl, combine coconut oil and essential oil.
3. Add the clay and baking soda mixture to the coconut and essential oil mixture.
4. Mix with a spoon until uniform and transfer into a container containing no metal.

Yield:
3 ounces

Preparation time:
15 minutes

Indications:
Clean teeth naturally while conditioning gums with this minty and refreshing toothpaste.

Usage:
Put a pea-sized amount on your toothbrush to brush teeth at least twice daily.

Storage:
Store in a cool, dry place for up to 6 months.

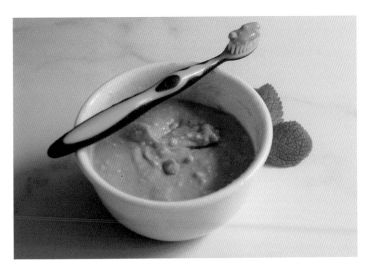

Toothpaste: It's minty fresh and cooling.

EXFOLIATING FACE WASH

Gentle, detoxifying, and exfoliating, this face wash will help slough away dead skin and draw out toxins and impurities to reveal brighter and more energized skin.

WHAT YOU'LL NEED:

- 2 teaspoons lavender flowers
- 1 teaspoon orange peel
- 1 cup melted unrefined coconut oil
- 1 teaspoon bentonite clay (don't use metal to scoop or store)
- 1 teaspoon Celtic sea salt (finely ground)

WHAT TO DO:

1. In an espresso grinder, grind lavender and orange peel to a fine consistency. The smell is so amazing!
2. In a separate pot, melt coconut oil over very low heat.
3. Add the orange peel and lavender along with the bentonite clay and sea salt directly into the melted coconut oil.
4. In a non-metal container (to avoid deactivating bentonite with metal), shake the oil with the exfoliants to combine and then pour into a storage container. I use an amber glass jar.
5. Refrigerate for 30 minutes, and it is ready to use.

Yield:
8 ounces

Preparation time:
45 minutes

Indications:
Brighten and exfoliate your skin with this gentle face wash.

Usage:
Mild enough for daily use. Apply a small amount and rub in a gentle circular motion. Use once daily.

Storage:
Store in a cool, dry place for up to 6 months.

COFFEE BODY SCRUB

If you are energized by the aroma of coffee, this scrub will make an excellent addition to your morning shower routine. Gently exfoliating and wonderfully fragrant with notes of vanilla and spices, this scrub is a wonderful post-soap or post–body wash choice.

WHAT YOU'LL NEED:

- 1½ cups brown sugar
- 2 tablespoons organic coffee grinds
- 1 cup coconut oil
- 1 teaspoon vanilla extract
- 1 teaspoon cinnamon
- 1 teaspoon vitamin E oil

WHAT TO DO:

1. Combine all ingredients in a bowl and mix with a spoon.

Yield:
12 ounces

Preparation time:
10 minutes

Indications:
Remove dead skin, soften, and plump skin with this coffee-based body scrub.

Usage:
Apply a small amount after washing to a sponge, brush, or washcloth and rub in a circular pattern. Rinse thoroughly.

Storage:
Store in a cool, dry place for up to 6 months.

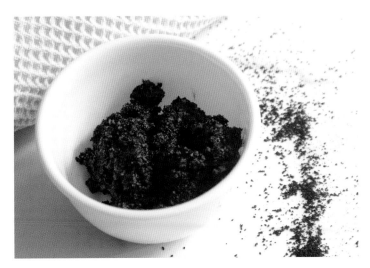

Coffee Body Scrub.

MOISTURIZING FACE MASK

In addition to being moisturizing, this mask formulation tones and restores the skin, balances pH levels, and brightens dull skin.

WHAT YOU'LL NEED:

- 2 tablespoons raw honey
- 1 teaspoon apple cider vinegar
- 1 tablespoon coconut oil

WHAT TO DO:

1. Combine honey and apple cider vinegar until thoroughly blended.
2. Add coconut oil and blend until smooth.

Yield:
1½ ounces

Preparation time:
5 minutes

Indications:
This mask naturally restores your skin's pH balance while detoxifying and sealing in moisture; it also gently exfoliates, revealing smooth, soft skin.

Usage:
Apply to a clean, dry face for 10 minutes, and then rinse off using a warm washcloth.

Storage:
Store in the refrigerator for up to 2 weeks.

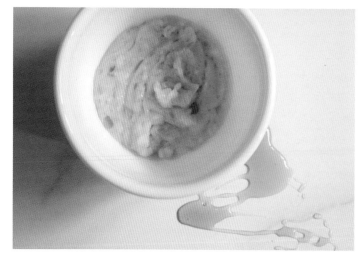

Moisturizing Face Mask.

HERBS AND SPICES
ZANZIBAR

Island off the Coast of Tanzania in Eastern Africa, Winter 2009

Zanzibar was a breathtaking cacophony of hues. My mouth was agape with wonder the moment the plane landed as I took in the greenest green, vibrantly bursting into dewy shadows depending on the direction of the sun.

My visit to Zanzibar was one of those last-minute and poorly planned trips that turned out to be one of my greatest decisions yet. We—some girlfriends and I—landed in Stone Town without a place to stay and without a clue. We assumed it would be easy enough to take a taxi from the airport and check into a hotel upon arrival—when you're in your twenties, who needs concrete plans?

As a result of our lack of planning, our taxi driver dropped us in the center of Stone Town. We had arrived, unknowingly, in the middle of the Sauti za Busara festival, a large festival celebrating music and musical artists across the continent of Africa that drew revelers from all over the world. Stone Town was crowded. Tourists had booked hotel rooms months in advance. Our introduction to the city, to Zanzibar, began on foot, flip-flops dragging over steeply inclined stone streets, rolling suitcases clattering as we trudged from one hotel to the next in the hopes of finding a place to stay.

It was the most spectacular place for us to be vagabonds. In the distance, the water shimmered, the setting sun casting an orange glow that framed the fishing boats that dotted the water. Fishermen cast their nets into the sea in the background, while, in the foreground, colorful compact vendor stalls were lined up and down the narrow streets selling kabobs, spices, and fruit. The ancient city, almost biblical in appearance, was aglow. Music echoed through the night.

We paused for water beneath a large acacia tree as the deep and stirring sound of the Islamic call to prayer rang out

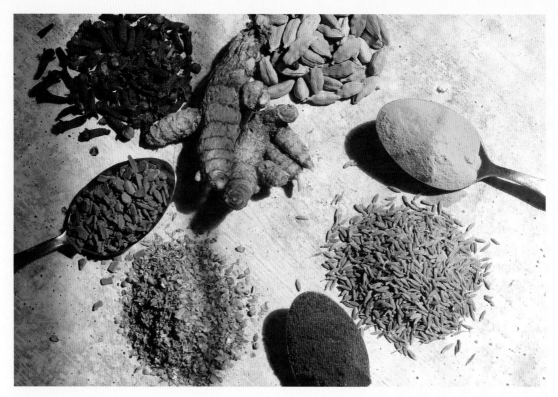

A variety of spices.

and everything came to a sudden stop. All music, all chatter muted. The echo seemed to emanate from every building in Stone Town, reverberating off the fishing boats docked in the still water. Colorful mats were unfurled all around us as people dropped to their knees in ritual prayer. Lost, tired, energized, in awe, we simply took it all in; even the elegant stray cats seemed to crouch and bow.

Moments later, as if being guided by an imaginary conductor, mats were rolled up, somewhere in the distance someone sneezed, a dog barked, the music started up again, and we continued our march, drifting from hotel to hotel in search of an opening.

At last, having climbed to the top of a steeply inclined, narrow street, behind a large stone gate, we found a room for the night in a private home at the suggestion of the man who had sold us our water. We had officially arrived.

In the days that followed, we maneuvered around the small island, leaving no nook unturned. Aside from delicious food, natural parks, and miles of untouched and pristine beaches, there was the music festival that we had unintentionally arrived in perfect time to enjoy. Zanzibar, it turned out, was a land of great hospitality. Our reckless lack of shelter was far from an issue, as we made new friends everywhere we went who put us up for days at a time in their homes. From ocean vistas to rain forest canopies, we traversed. The rich musk of the earth and the fragrance of fresh rain combined with the sweet crispy smoke of a wood-burning stove. This scent followed us from the sprawling spice plantations inland to the coral forests and even the white sand beaches along the coast.

One of my favorite haunts was the large spice market in Stone Town, an Ayurvedic practitioner's dream, where I became a regular. Walking the cobblestone streets, with a flowing muslin scarf loosely covering my head and shoulders and the scent of ginger, cardamom and clove heavy in the air, I was transported to another time and place. I didn't want to leave. Every turn down the narrow and congested pathways revealed a new treasure. I encountered the rich and fragrantly layered vanilla pods produced on the island. It was my first time really experiencing vanilla outside of the extract I'd purchase in the grocery store in the amber bottles. There were round balls of nutmeg, grounding and fragrant, and shiny red chilies dried in the sun ready to be ground into spice. I also saw large, gnarled roots of turmeric and ginger. My senses danced as the spices I learned about in my Ayurvedic course came boldly to life.

I peered shamelessly into barrels of freshly harvested spices: containers of whole black pepper and mustard seed, star anise, and peppers of every shape, size, and color. I was so used to the finely ground, prepackaged versions of these spices. I had considered myself so knowledgeable about spices, their properties and applications, but here, beneath the canopy of the central market, I realized how little I knew.

"Mambo," I would call out in greeting, an enthusiastic smile on my face. I had so many questions. My new friend Abdul, an artist from Kenya I had met at the festival, had patiently taught me a few key phrases in Swahili. Though everyone for the most part spoke English, I found people were much more likely to engage in a conversation with you in English if you first made the effort to connect with them in Swahili or Arabic. Having never heard either language spoken until touching down in Zanzibar, my pronunciations were awkward; my flailing tongue felt clumsy in my mouth. But, determined, I prattled away, oftentimes to the curious amusement of the vendors I would eventually win over and form a connection with; from there,

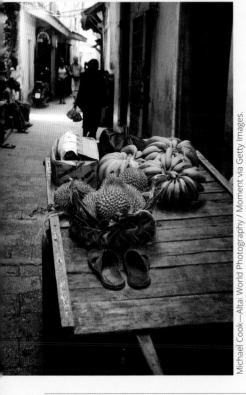

Michael Cook—Altai World Photography / Moment via Getty Images.

JohanSjolander/E+ via Getty Images.

Stone Town, Zanzibar.

At left: Fruit for sale, Stone Town, Zanzibar.

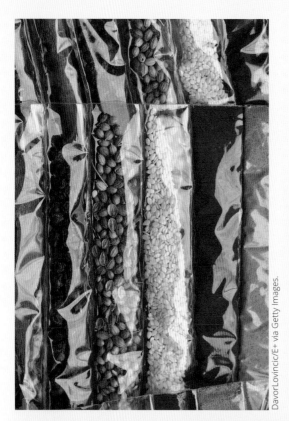

DavorLovincic/E+ via Getty Images.

Spices at market.

Below: Black pepper and turmeric.

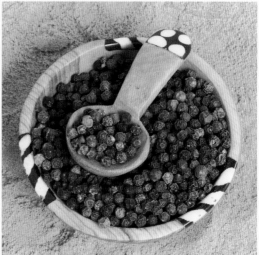

Tuul & Bruno Morandi / The Image Bank via Getty Images.

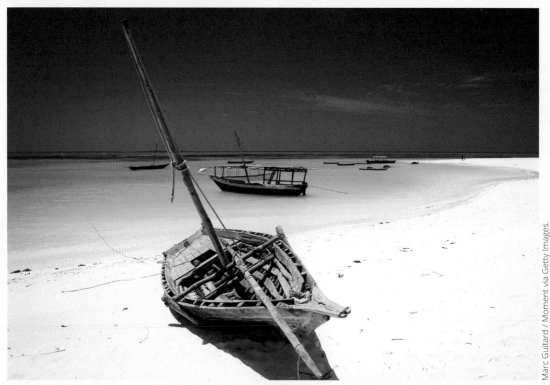

Marc Guitard / Moment via Getty Images.

Dhow boat, Zanzibar.

I was often invited not only to smell and touch but also to taste. *"A-salamu Aaay-kum! Wa-alaykum salaam"* ("Peace be with you and also with you") is how my visits to each stall would begin and end. Off I would go to the next shop, with my collection of bags, new friends, and packages growing larger.

My spice adventures culminated in a trip to the countryside in the north region to a working plantation and a daylong trek through the mountains to identify herbs and spices. We departed Stone Town early one morning by bus and rode past the boundary of the city into the vibrant green countryside. We were let off near the opening of a small village at the base of a mountain. Here we met our guide, who led us on a hike up the mountain as we stopped to identify spices and herbs along the way.

With my bare hands, I uncovered turmeric root. The soil, black and volcanic, gave way to my eager fingers as the astringent, orange root tumbled into my hands. There was ginger root, peppery, bulbous, and eager. My basket became heavy, bearing the gnarled weight of the robust roots. We picked vanilla beans—shiny, black, shriveled pods, revealing the richest, sweetly scented vanilla I'd ever encountered. We found green cardamom pods that we'd crack open with our teeth, sucking on the spicy seeds until they sweetened our breath. Then we came across pepper, cayenne, cinnamon—the world seemed so colorful, alive, and fertile. I was seduced by the aromas and tastes, the colors and sounds.

During that mountain trek, our guide and a group of local women taught us how to prepare food, oils, and skin concoctions using the spices we'd helped harvest. I could barely contain myself. My mind was in overdrive, recalling lessons from my Ayurvedic studies. Everything clicked into place as I learned about the herbal traditions of this remarkable eastern African nation. My heart swelled and danced as memories, extracted from the aromas, rose to the surface.

After handing over our harvest to a group of women from the village, we were treated that evening to the most phenomenal dinner of spiced flatbreads, curried lentils, grilled vegetables, seasoned beans, spiced coffee, and fragrant tandoori-style meat. We dined in the open air, seated barefoot on colorful blankets beneath the constellation of stars. I could have stayed on that mountain in the countryside throughout eternity. The island of Zanzibar was a door into a complex and colorful world, a door into myself.

Reluctant to leave, it's a wonder I made it through customs and back onto the island of Manhattan with all of my goodies intact. When I returned to my tiny East Village apartment, the first thing I did was create a treasure trove out of my spice drawer incorporating the flavors, aromas, and colors from Zanzibar into my relatively predictable collection of herbs, salts, and peppers.

Ancient people have always understood that the power of spices, minerals, herbs, and flowers extended beyond their consumable benefits. In the same sense that spices were used to preserve meat, fish, and, well, mummies, they were also used on living, breathing, human beings to treat skin conditions, detoxify the skin, and promote and preserve beauty. Ancient Egyptians used such spices as cinnamon, cardamom, black pepper, mustard seed, and ginger medicinally as well as to beautify their skin. Cleopatra herself was known to rub Dead Sea salt over her body as a natural exfoliator and a way to replenish minerals. Frankincense and myrrh resins were used to preserve and maintain healthy skin. Ancient Egyptians used sugaring techniques for hair removal as well as henna, a plant-derived dye from the henna tree, to dye their fingernails yellow and orange, which helped condition nails and promote healthy growth.

In India, where much of the knowledge from ancient Egypt was disseminated, contributing to Ayurvedic practices, turmeric was and still is rubbed onto the faces of young brides as a way to clear blemishes and inflammation, ignite a golden glow, and promote beauty. Cinnamon is also used directly on the skin to fight blemishes, exfoliate, and promote healthy circulation.

In England, dried, crushed rose petals were used to moisturize the skin and scalp. Thyme was used to clean the scalp and stimulate hair growth, and dried lavender was used to heal inflammation and burns.

There are so many different ways to use spices and dried herbs directly on the skin or in skin formulations. Our earliest human ancestors understood the benefits of this practice in a quite intimate and remarkable way. They understood nature and how to adjust their routines to the seasons, and they knew what natural ingredients to use to create internal and external balance. The answers can all be found in nature. Nature, not the lab, creates some of the most effective and pleasurable skin formulations. I'll outline some of my favorite recipes in the following pages.

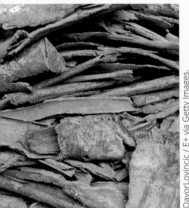

Cinnamon bark.

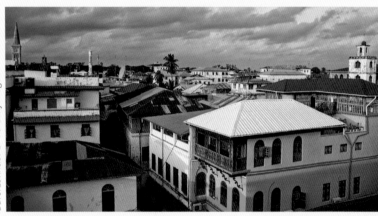

Stone Town, Zanzibar.

DavorLovincic / E+ via Getty Images.

Photography by Jeremy Villasis, Philippines / Moment via Getty Images.

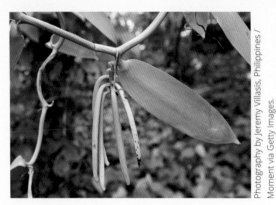

Vanilla pods.

Photography by Jeremy Villasis, Philippines / Moment via Getty Images.

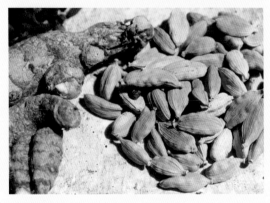

Cardamom and turmeric.

GINGER/LEMON SALT SCRUB

This is a fresh and invigorating full-body scrub that effectively promotes healthy circulation while brightening and softening skin.

WHAT YOU'LL NEED:

- 1 cup coarse sea salt
- 2 tablespoons shaved lemon rind (dried)
- 2 tablespoons ginger
- ½ cup coconut oil (softened)

WHAT TO DO:

1. In a bowl, combine sea salt, lemon rind, and ginger.
2. If your coconut oil is hard, soften it by running the jar under warm water. Add the softened coconut oil to the mixture and combine.
3. Add to a storage jar.

Yield:
10 ounces

Preparation time:
5 minutes

Indications:
Invigorating and stimulating, this full-body scrub will clear away dead skin and help increase circulation.

Usage:
Apply a small amount to your body after washing. Massage in a circular motion and rinse fully.

Storage:
Store in a cool, dry place for up to 6 months.

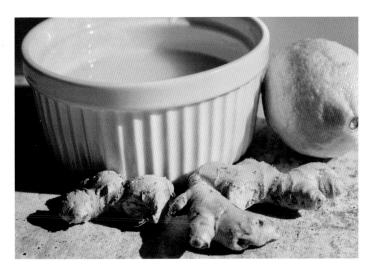

Ginger/Lemon Salt Scrub.

GOLDEN MILK SUGAR SCRUB

Reminiscent of a soothing cup of golden milk, this grounding full-body scrub is antibacterial and moisturizing, making it ideal for calming everything from nerves and inflamed skin to acne and fungal conditions.

WHAT YOU'LL NEED:

- 1 cup organic brown sugar
- 1 teaspoon turmeric
- 1 teaspoon cardamom
- ½ teaspoon cinnamon
- ¼ cup coconut oil
- ¼ cup coconut cream

WHAT TO DO:

1. In a bowl, combine the brown sugar, turmeric, cardamom, and cinnamon.
2. In a separate bowl, combine the coconut oil and coconut cream until uniform in texture.
3. Add the coconut oil and cream mixture to the brown sugar mixture.
4. Once thoroughly mixed, transfer to a storage container.

Yield:
One 10-ounce jar

Preparation time:
10 minutes

Indications:
This sugar scrub is anti-inflammatory and moisturizing.

Usage:
Warm in palms before putting on body. Apply a small amount to body after washing. Massage in a circular motion to gently moisturize, nourish, and calm skin.

Storage:
Store in the refrigerator for up to 6 months.

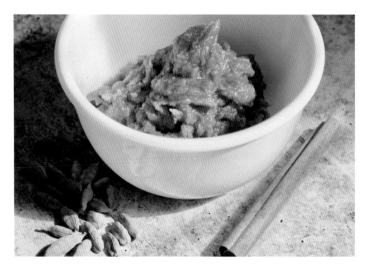

Golden Milk Sugar Scrub.

BRIGHTENING FACIAL SCRUB

This scrub, designed specifically for the delicate skin of the face, gently brightens to reveal a vibrant and rejuvenated appearance. Antimicrobial and antibacterial, the scrub will also help pacify acne.

WHAT YOU'LL NEED:

- ¼ cup organic brown sugar
- 1 tablespoon finely ground dried orange peel
- 2 teaspoons dried ground oregano
- ¼ cup raw honey

WHAT TO DO:

1. Combine brown sugar, orange peel, and oregano.
2. Add honey to the sugar mixture.
3. Place in a storage container.

Yield:
4 ounces

Preparation time:
5 minutes

Indications:
This facial scrub is brightening, cleansing, detoxifying, and purifying.

Usage:
After washing, apply a small amount to the facial skin. Massage in a circular pattern before rinsing thoroughly. Use 2–3 times a week.

Storage:
Store in the refrigerator for up to 6 weeks.

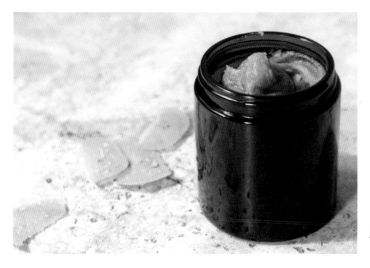

Brightening Facial Scrub.

47

FRANKINCENSE AND MYRRH BATH BOMBS

Luxuriate in the tub with these fizzy and aromatic bath bombs. Frankincense and myrrh offer grounding and soothing qualities while delicately working to restore and regenerate skin, guarding against premature aging.

WHAT YOU'LL NEED:

- 1 cup baking soda
- ½ cup citric acid
- ½ cup Epsom salts
- ¾ cup cornstarch
- 1 teaspoon ground frankincense resin
- 1 teaspoon ground myrrh resin
- 2 tablespoons argan oil
- 3 teaspoons witch hazel
- Bath bomb mold or muffin tin

WHAT TO DO:

1. In a bowl, combine baking soda, citric acid, Epsom salts, cornstarch, and ground frankincense and myrrh.
2. In a separate bowl, combine argan oil and witch hazel.
3. Add the argan oil and witch hazel mixture to the dry ingredient mixture a teaspoon at a time until slowly blended.
4. Grease bath bomb molds or muffin tin mold with argan oil and press the mixture firmly into the mold.
5. Refrigerate and leave for 48 hours until hardened and expanded.
6. Remove from tray.

Yield:
Depends on mold used

Preparation time:
2 days

Indications:
These fragrant, calming bath bombs detoxify, exfoliate, and moisturize skin.

Usage:
Draw a warm bath, add your bath bomb, and soak.

Storage:
Store in a plastic bag and keep in the refrigerator for up to 2 weeks.

THYME HERBAL BATH

Imagine soaking in a giant tea cup—that's what this thyme herbal bath experience is like. Beautifully aromatic and uplifting, this bath blend detoxifies, draws out impurities from the skin, and relaxes tired muscles.

WHAT YOU'LL NEED:

- 1 cup Epsom salts
- ¼ cup dried thyme
- 2 tablespoon dried hibiscus flower
- 1 tablespoon dried chamomile flower

WHAT TO DO:

1. Combine ingredients in a storage jar and mix until fully blended.

Yield:
16 ounces

Preparation time:
5 minutes

Indications:
This deeply detoxifying, warming, and invigorating bath soak is excellent for tired muscles, inflammation in the joints, and clogged pores.

Usage:
Draw a warm bath and add between ¼ cup and 1 cup of the mixture (as desired) to the bath water. Sit in the bath until the water becomes lukewarm. Dry skin and follow up with a moisturizer.

Storage:
Store in a jar in a cool, dry location.

SPICY CHAI BATH SALTS

Refreshing and nourishing, this grounding bath is profoundly detoxifying and stimulating. You will emerge like new and smelling like a chai latte.

WHAT YOU'LL NEED:

- 2 tablespoons sweet almond oil
- 10 drops cardamom essential oil
- 5 drops clove essential oil
- 5 drops cinnamon essential oil
- 1 cup Epsom salts
- 1 cup Himalayan pink salt
- ¼ cup baking soda
- 2 tablespoons ground cardamom
- 1 tablespoon ground dried orange peel
- 1 tablespoon ground ginger
- 2 teaspoons ground dried clove
- 2 teaspoons ground dried cinnamon
- ¼ teaspoon ground turmeric

WHAT TO DO:

1. In a small bowl, blend the sweet almond oil and essential oils.
2. In a larger bowl or in a storage jar that is at least 20 ounces, combine the Epsom and pink salt until uniform.
3. Add the baking soda and mix until thoroughly blended.
4. One by one, add and blend in the ground cardamom, dried orange peel, ginger, clove, cinnamon, and turmeric.
5. Pour the sweet almond and essential oil mixture over the dry salt and herb mixture.
6. Mix until the salts take on a gritty and slightly moist overall consistency.

Yield:
20 ounces

Preparation time:
20 minutes

Indications:
These bath salts moisturize the skin while providing anti-inflammatory and anti-aging benefits.

Usage:
Draw a warm bath and add a ¼ cup scoop to the warm bath water. Soak for as long as you'd like.

Storage:
Store in a mason jar or amber or cobalt jar for up to a year in a cool, dry place.

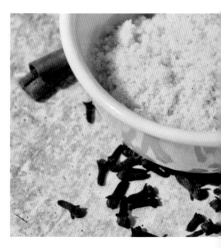

Spicy Chai Bath Salts.

CARRIER OILS
JAMAICA

Island in the Caribbean Sea, Summer 2013

We were up high in the dense green mountainous outskirts of Negril, Jamaica. Our temporary home was a former banana plantation turned nature reserve and guest resort, for which I was working on a travel article. The air clung heavy and humid. In the distance, a surprisingly still, sparkling blue ocean beckoned, but the dense overcast sky told a different story. It was monsoon season. A few days into our stay on the massive plantation property, the sky opened up. Rain drummed down, turning the tin roof covering our bungalow into a percussion instrument. My husband Mark and I spent an entire week indoors with a restless one-year-old.

During this time, I put the finishing touches on my article so that after the rains, when nature burst forth with resplendent glory, I was able to engage without distraction. The beauty of the mountainous western coast of Jamaica is astonishing. Hummingbirds danced like furious, colorful fairies around wild ginger flowers. Peacocks walked the ixora-studded paths that wound through the property connecting bungalows to beach paths, hiking trails, and the one restaurant.

On the lagoon side of the 100-acre property, bullfrogs croaked as crocodiles, silent and stealthy, cut through the water without so much as a splash.

We were in our own little bubble of paradise. Away from the popular resorts, the busy towns, and the hustle and bustle of Negril and other tourists, we worked intimately with a local guide, a steward of the reserve, and joined him for crocodile feedings and herb walks. Winston, our guide, led Mark and me, with our

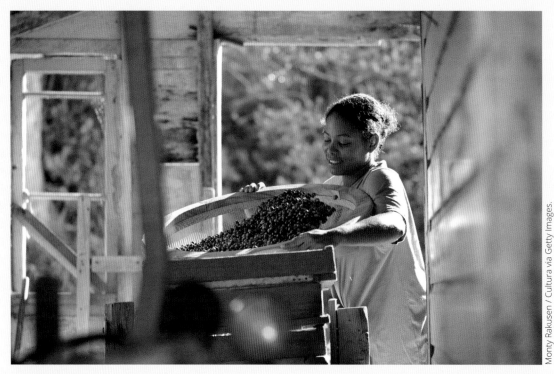

Monty Rakusen / Cultura via Getty Images.

Jamaican coffee plantation.

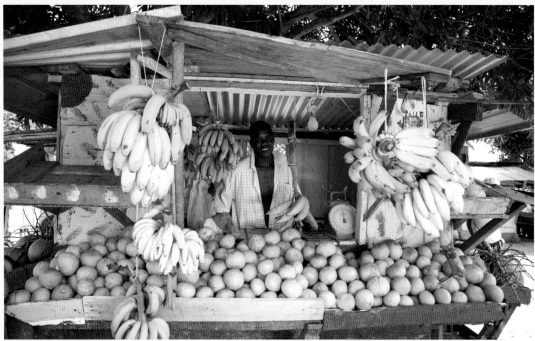

Buena Vista Images / Photodisc via Getty Images.

Jamaican fruit vendor.

one-year-old son harnessed to my back in his carrier, through murky bogs, past banyan trees, and into old plantation fields and wild herb gardens. Winston was a passionate environmentalist, and in a series of inspired, long-winded sermons, he educated us about the conservation of vulnerable species and his favorite topic: the local roots and medicinal flowers that called the mountains home. Every afternoon was a new adventure.

Part historian, part naturalist, part encyclopedia, Winston gave us a thorough and fascinating introduction to the wild herbs of Jamaica and their uses by locals. Jamaica has such a rich herbal tradition—a tradition that can be traced back to indigenous inhabitants like the Taino Indians, who had highly developed agricultural and medicinal systems. When enslaved Africans were brought to Jamaica, they brought with them complex herbal knowledge from their home countries, and over time, through intermarriage and cultural diffusion, they learned from and added to the natural healing practices that were already prevalent. With the introduction of Indians from South Asia, who brought with them to Jamaica Ayurvedic herbal traditions, Jamaica became a melting pot and developed a solid and unshakable culture of herbal folk medicine, one that is fully intact to this day.

Winston was a patient and disciplined teacher. He taught us to forage thyme and basil, wild ginger, and anise. We examined whole nutmeg and vanilla pods, which took my memory back to my sojourn to Zanzibar. I saw ackee plants up close, gathered jackfruit, picked burgundy sorrel leaves, and nursed the sap from large, fat aloe vera plants.

It was on one such walk that I was introduced to something that would become a staple in my bath and beauty formulations. Winston produced a handful of brown and gray seeds with black specks. The seeds came from a burgundy-leafed plant with the most stunning scarlet pods. Within the pods were the seeds. I had met the castor bean plant, and Winston made it his business to share with me the wonders of its beloved by-product, black castor oil.

Not all castor oil is the same. Through my Ayurvedic studies, I had worked with castor oil before. Castor oil was an Ayurvedic remedy for constipation, and I had suggested that many a client use castor oil packs or rub castor oil on the soles of their feet to stimulate their bowels. I even had some personal experience with castor oil. When I was pregnant and carrying well past my due date, my midwife ordered me to consume castor oil to stimulate contractions. It was far from pleasant to drink tablespoonfuls of the thick and, in my opinion, shoe-polish-flavored oil. I gagged, I wretched, and I swore to never go near the stuff again. The fact that there was a black castor oil specific to Jamaica that reportedly worked wonders for the hair, however, was news to me.

When it came to the topic of castor oil in particular, Winston's eyes lit up. He went into detail, talking about how he had used the oil on his hair when he had locks and how his mother used it on her hair, which was well past her waist—a result of the castor oil, according to him.

After a few hikes through the mountains with Winston, I wanted to try black castor oil for myself. I had been taught to extract the jellybean-like seeds from the pod, but I didn't have the actual oil for context. To get the oil, I'd have to leave the reserve and go into Negril, the closest town, to buy some Jamaican black castor oil at a local market.

The town of Negril was busy and intense. We took a taxi and were dropped off near a congested cluster of shops. After a few quick rounds of browsing, I emerged with a bottle. We had lunch at Rick's Café with a view of the cliff jumpers before heading back to the reserve.

The next morning, I opened the bottle. I rubbed it on my hair, I rubbed it on my skin, I used it on my one-year-old's eczema-prone knees and elbows, and I used it to refresh my husband's beard. It was lovely. Black castor oil was thick, luxurious, and moisturizing. My hair shone, my husband's beard glistened, and my son's eczema patches seemed to be placated. There was just one problem: the smell. I couldn't get past the heavy aroma, which reminded me of the time when I gagged down several tablespoonfuls in an attempt to induce contractions. It wasn't just me; my husband Mark also commented on the aroma, as he kept getting strong whiffs from his beard.

When two weeks later I made it back to my Brooklyn apartment, where I was reunited with a working internet connection, I did my own research. In addition to learning about the curative properties of black castor oil, I found that if I blended the carrier oil with peppermint or tea tree essential oil, I didn't notice the smell, and I was able to apply the oil as liberally as I wanted without it making my stomach churn.

As it turned out (and I had expected nothing less), Winston was on to something, and here's why: Castor oil comes from the seeds of the castor plant, the wispy eggplant purple stalk with the curious spiky bulbous pods that I'd encountered on the reserve. The type of castor oil that I was used to, clear and thick, was made by pressing fresh seeds. Jamaican black castor oil was unique in that it was expressed from seeds that had first been roasted, pounded, and boiled. This process of roasting the seeds produced ash—hence the black color of the oil. This is where the magic apparently lay in the Jamaican castor oil variety. The black ash altered the pH balance of the castor oil, causing it to become more alkaline, in turn remarkably enhancing the healing properties of the castor oil.

As a powerfully curative carrier oil, there are of course numerous uses for Jamaican black castor oil, but I was most interested in its benefits to the hair, specifically for softening and moisturizing, creating shine, and stimulating thick growth. Applying castor oil to the scalp and smoothing it over the hair shaft helps create thick, soft, shiny locks. You can also use it to encourage thick and bold eyebrow growth. Black castor oil is likewise used to treat baldness. How? It's in the science.

Black castor oil contains ricinoleic acid, which helps increase blood circulation to the scalp and enliven hair follicles. Nutrients are more efficiently transmitted to the hair, encouraging healthy and robust growth. The ricinoleic acid in Jamaican black castor oil also helps balance the pH of the scalp and is antibacterial, antifungal, and anti-inflammatory. This helps fight against dandruff, keeps the hair clean and bacteria-free naturally, and keeps the scalp free of irritating skin infections that can act as an impediment to growth. These qualities also make black castor oil

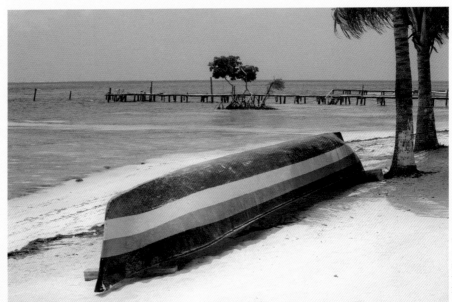

Boat on Jamaican beach.

Jzabloski/E+ via Getty Images.

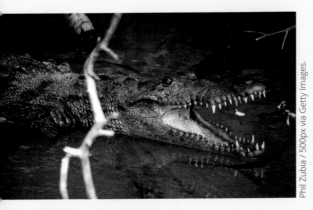

Alligator on mangroves.

Phil Zubia / 500px via Getty Images.

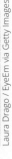

At river's edge.

Laura Drago / EyeEm via Getty Images.

an effective treatment for certain types of eczema. In addition, Jamaican black castor oil is full of antioxidants that support keratin growth in hair, which in turn strengthens hair, resulting in smoother, softer, and less frizzy locks. Keratin helps strengthen the roots of hair, which can result in reduced hair loss. With this new awareness, Jamaican black castor oil became one of my favorite carrier oils.

Carrier oils by definition are oils that are used to "carry" or dilute essential oils in preparations. These oils are typically cold pressed from the nuts, seeds, or kernels of a plant and serve as a base so that essential oils can be safely diluted and applied onto the skin. Most essential oils should not be applied directly to the skin because they are so powerful and concentrated that the result would be extreme epidermal irritation. This is why carrier oils are so important. Some examples of carrier oils are jojoba, olive, castor, coconut, safflower, almond, and avocado, to name a few.

Carrier oils with a mild aroma are typically preferred, as they will not interact with or distort the aroma of the essential oils they are being blended with. Carrier oils are like the ocean. Deep, dense, and nutrient rich, they hold space for all the other liquids, oils, herbs, and ingredients that make up the blends we use for bath and body products. Derived from vegetables, fruits, seeds, and nuts, they can be chosen (depending on the desired outcome) for their cosmetic and healing properties. Carrier oils can be used for skin care, hair care, oil infusions, cosmetics, aromatherapy, and healing and medicinal products, as well as cleaning products.

When dealing with the body, carrier oils tend to be used primarily for diluting essential oils. Since essential oils are heavily concentrated, placing a few drops of essential oils in a base of carrier oils helps ensure that the use of essential oils is safe.

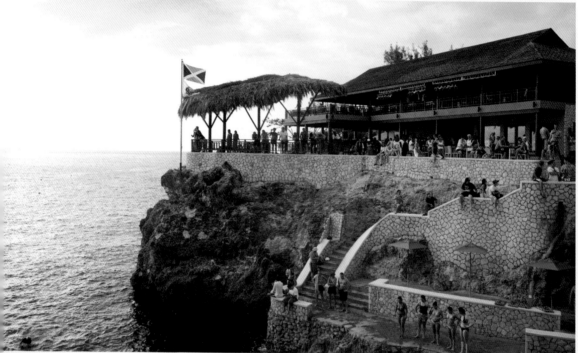

Buena Vista Images / Stone via Getty Images.

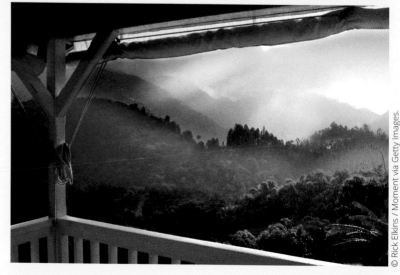

Above: The cliffs in Negril, Jamaica.

Sunrise over the mountains.

© Rick Elkins / Moment via Getty Images.

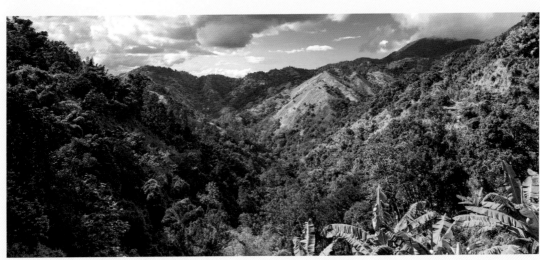
Blue Mountains of Jamaica.

TYPES OF OILS

Cold-pressed oils are the most natural oils that you can buy. The integrity of the oil is almost wholly preserved through the process of cold pressing. When an oil is cold pressed, oil is extracted through a process of pressing, which is done with a machine press that exceeds no more than 120 degrees Fahrenheit. Cold-pressed oil is "raw" if it's heated no more than 110 degrees Fahrenheit. Cold-pressed oils have the highest percentage of nutrients.

Expeller-pressed oils are slightly more processed than cold-pressed oils in that the oils are pressed at a temperature a touch higher than cold pressed (120 degrees to 200 degrees Fahrenheit). The heat during this process can somewhat compromise the quality of the oil, depleting some of its essential nutrients.

Solvent-extracted oils use a solvent like hexane to extract the oils. Trace solvent particles can be found in the oil after this process, while nutrients and fatty acids are also destroyed. Solvent-extracted oils are the least natural oils that you can buy.

In addition to the way in which an oil is extracted, oils can be unrefined or refined.

Unrefined oils are oils that are barely altered after the oil is pressed. Through this process, a screen is used to filter out whatever small particles may be mixed into the batch of oil. This process doesn't compromise nutrients, vitamins, and fatty acids, as there is no heat involved. The highest-quality oils are unrefined.

Refined oils are oils that are processed after they have been pressed. The process of refining oils destroys the majority of nutrients. Refining oils is popular because the procedure helps increase shelf life. During refinement, colors and odors are removed using high heat, freezing, bleaching, and deodorization. This process destroys vital nutrients.

Another area of oil confusion lies in understanding the difference between extra virgin and virgin oil. These designations are typically reserved for olive oils.

Extra virgin oil is pressed one time and is the purest form.

Virgin oil is pressed multiple times, which dilutes nutrients and purity.

COMMON CARRIER OILS
(For Cosmetic Use and Essential Oil Blends)

COCONUT OIL

- Rich in antioxidants
- Antifungal
- Anti-inflammatory
- Antibacterial
- 50% lauric acid (assists as a preservative for a long shelf life)
- Moisturizing

OLIVE OIL

- 75% oleic acid (potent anti-inflammatory)
- Nongreasy
- Won't clog skin pores or leave hair greasy
- Moisturizing

JOJOBA OIL

- Anti-inflammatory
- Light
- Mimics closely the body's sebum (skin oil)
- Absorbs into the skin without a trace

SWEET ALMOND OIL

- Rich in vitamin E
- Antioxidant
- Regenerative
- Promotes new skin cells
- Locks in moisture
- Great for aging skin
- Moisturizes dry skin

ARGAN OIL
(*From the Moroccan Argan Tree*)

- Anti-aging
- Promotes hair growth
- High in vitamins A and E
- Helps repair UV damage
- Reduces appearance of stretch marks and scars

AVOCADO OIL

- Luxurious and thick
- Great for anti-aging
- High in palmitoleic acid (a type of fatty acid found naturally in human fatty tissues just under the skin)
- Great for mature skin
- High in vitamins A, D, and E
- Anti-inflammatory

GRAPESEED OIL

- High in antioxidants
- Rich in minerals
- High in vitamin E
- High in linoleic acid
- Antiseptic
- Mild astringent

MARULA OIL

- High in antioxidants
- Softens and moisturizes skin
- Supports aging and sun-damaged skin
- Pacifies acne
- Rich in essential fatty acids
- Reduces scarring

MORINGA OIL

- 70% oleic acid
- Strengthens cell membranes and repairs damaged cells
- Rich in antioxidants
- Anti-inflammatory
- High in vitamin A
- Boosts collagen and accelerates wound healing
- Protects from UV and environmental damage

APRICOT KERNEL OIL

- Light oil
- Softens skin
- Nongreasy

CASTOR OIL
(*From the Seed of the Castor Bean Plant*)

- Kills bacteria
- Increases white blood cells
- Antifungal
- Antiviral
- High in ricinoleic acid that enhances immunity through stimulating the lymphatic system, which helps the body detoxify and improves circulation

BLACK SEED OIL
(*From the Seed of the Caraway Plant*)

- 50% linoleic acid
- Rich in thymoquinone, thymohydroquinone, and thymol (antibacterial, antifungal, analgesic, and anti-inflammatory)
- Restores hair loss
- Reduces the appearance of scars and blemishes
- Boosts immunity

EVENING PRIMROSE OIL

- Improves hormonal balance
- High in linoleic and gamma-linoleic acid (anti-inflammatory)

NEEM OIL

- Eliminates parasites
- Insecticide (due to azadirachtin)
- Stimulates collagen production
- Reduces the appearance of old scars
- Promotes healing and softening of skin

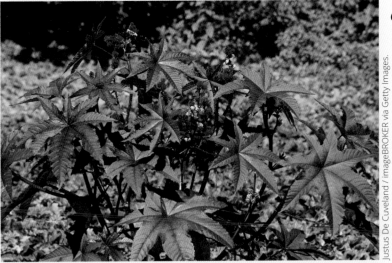

Castor oil plant.

Justus De Cuveland / imageBROKER via Getty Images.

HEMP SEED OIL

- High in linoleic and alpha-linolenic acid
- Anti-inflammatory
- Skin regenerating
- Anti-aging
- Natural pain reliever
- Nongreasy

ROSEHIP OIL

- Boosts collagen
- Improves skin elasticity
- Anti-aging
- Reduces stretch marks
- High in linoleic and alpha-linolenic acid
- High in vitamins A and E

FLAXSEED OIL

- Highest concentration of alpha-linoleic acid among vegetable-based carrier oils
- Powerful anti-inflammatory properties

TAMANU OIL

- Skin rejuvenating
- Rapid wound healing
- Encourages cellular regeneration
- Tissue growth
- Antioxidant
- Reduces scars, stretch marks, and age spots
- Seals in moisture

There are so many different ways to use carrier oils in skin and hair formulations. I'll outline some of my favorite recipes in the following pages.

ANTI-AGING FACIAL SERUM

This is a great daytime serum designed to ward off the signs of aging. Wear under your moisturizer, sunscreen, or makeup. Contains light UV protection.

WHAT YOU'LL NEED:

- 2 tablespoons tamanu oil
- 10 drops frankincense essential oil
- 5 drops lavender essential oil

WHAT TO DO:

1. This mixture can be combined directly in your storage container. I recommend a glass bottle with a dropper lid.
2. Fill your bottle with the tamanu oil first, and then add the essential oils.
3. Shake gently to combine.

Yield:
1 ounce

Preparation time:
5 minutes

Indications:
Combat the signs of aging with this intensive cellular-regenerating facial serum.

Usage:
After washing, apply to face and neck twice daily. Makeup and creams can be worn on top.

Storage:
Store in a cool, dry place out of direct sunlight.

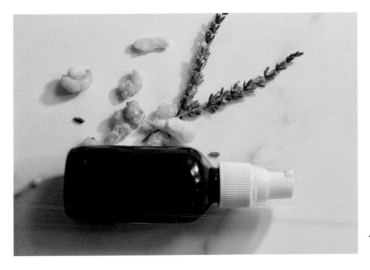

Anti-aging Facial Serum.

SKIN-SMOOTHING FACIAL SERUM

Keep your skin youthful and fresh with this skin-smoothing facial serum. Perfect for sensitive skin, this formula can be used twice daily after washing and toning.

WHAT YOU'LL NEED:

- 1 ounce rosehip oil
- 1 ounce hemp seed oil
- 10 drops geranium essential oil
- 5 drops ylang ylang essential oil

WHAT TO DO:

1. This mixture can be created directly in the storage container. I recommend a glass bottle with a dropper lid.
2. Combine the rosehip oil and hemp oil.
3. Add the geranium and ylang ylang essential oils and shake gently to blend.

Yield:
2 ounces

Preparation time:
5 minutes

Indications:
This light and aromatic serum plumps and smooths the skin.

Usage:
After washing, apply to face and neck. Creams and makeup can be worn on top.

Storage:
Store in a cool, dry place out of direct sunlight for up to a year.

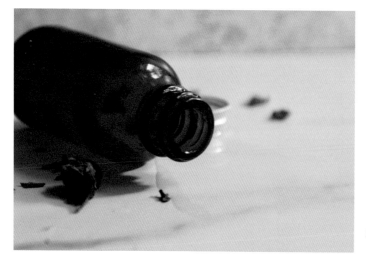

Skin-Smoothing Facial Serum.

SCAR-REDUCING OIL

This concentrated oil formula will smooth, retexture, and reduce the appearance of scars.

WHAT YOU'LL NEED:

- 1 ounce moringa oil
- 1 ounce sweet almond oil
- 10 drops helichrysum essential oil
- 10 drops carrot seed essential oil

WHAT TO DO:

1. This mixture can be created directly in the storage container. I recommend a glass bottle with a dropper lid.
2. Combine moringa oil and sweet almond oil.
3. Add the helichrysum and carrot seed essential oils and shake gently to blend.

Yield:
2 ounces

Preparation time:
5 minutes

Indications:
Regular use of this oil as a spot treatment may greatly reduce the appearance of scars.

Usage:
After washing, apply using your fingertip or a cotton ball, as a spot treatment, directly on the scar or area that needs work.

Storage:
Store in a cool, dry place for up to a year.

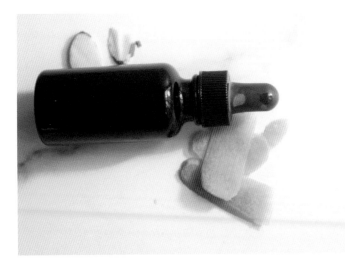

Scar-Reducing Oil.

HAIR-GROWTH OIL

Stimulate hair growth naturally with this oil formula, which is designed to clear the scalp and increase circulation to reveal healthy, long locks.

WHAT YOU'LL NEED:

- 1½ ounces black castor oil
- ½ ounce neem oil
- 10 drops lemongrass essential oil
- 10 drops lavender essential oil

WHAT TO DO:

1. This mixture can be created directly in the storage container. I recommend a glass bottle with a dropper lid.
2. Combine black castor oil and neem oil.
3. Add the lemongrass and lavender essential oils and shake gently to blend.

Yield:
2 ounces

Preparation time:
5 minutes

Indications:
This oil naturally cleanses, detoxifies, and exfoliates the scalp, making way for healthy, thick, uninhibited hair growth.

Usage:
Apply directly to the scalp before grooming, using a glass bottle with a dropper attachment, and massage into scalp using fingertips.

Storage:
Store in a cool, dry place for up to an hour.

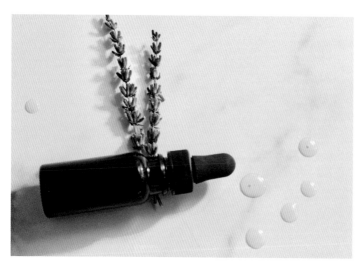

Hair-Growth Oil.

MOISTURIZING BODY OIL

Like a liquid lotion, this body oil formula will moisturize skin while combating signs of aging.

WHAT YOU'LL NEED:

- 2 ounces jojoba oil
- 2 ounces apricot oil
- 15 drops sandalwood essential oil
- 10 drops myrrh essential oil

WHAT TO DO:

1. This mixture can be created directly in the storage container.
2. Combine jojoba oil and apricot oil.
3. Add the sandalwood and myrrh essential oils.

Yield:
4 ounces

Preparation time:
5 minutes

Indications:
This light and nongreasy body oil absorbs easily, leaving behind soft and balanced skin.

Usage:
Apply a dime-sized amount in your hand and smooth over body either after a shower or whenever you need it.

Storage:
Store in a cool, dry place for up to a year.

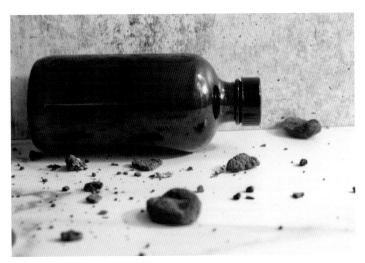

Moisturizing Body Oil.

FLORAL WATERS
PORTUGAL

Southern Europe, Summer 2013

Right before my oldest son turned two, my sister, N'Djamena, and I took a trip to Portugal. It was one last international trip before I'd soon have to pay full price for the little guy to fly. One final hurrah before he entered toddlerhood and would no longer be content to view the world calmly from the vantage point of his carrier strapped to my chest.

After having lived in Mozambique, a country still emerging from beneath the colonial weight of Portuguese influence, I was interested in learning more about this small country in Europe that had such an impact on my favorite place in the world: Inhambane, Mozambique.

During my southern African travels, I had met many Portuguese people and had learned to speak Portuguese and was comfortably conversational. I had also developed a fondness for Portuguese food and flavors, especially the delectable breads and the unforgettably feisty piri piri pepper sauce.

N'Djamena, a New Yorker to her core who worked in the fashion industry, was over the moon at the prospect of exploring Lisbon's art, textile, and design scene. During our flight to Portugal, she flipped through Portuguese magazines and created lists of places that she wanted to visit. Since I merely wanted to eat and wine taste my way through the city, and maybe take in some Fado music, N'Djamena was in charge of our itinerary.

Lisbon was stunning. There was a vibrant yet settled artistic air about the city. Architecturally stately and ancient, colorful Moorish tiles glistened off buildings. Old churches, graying and cracked from centuries of sun and rain, rose over the terra-cotta-tiled roofs of residential buildings and cafés. Like a prim lady,

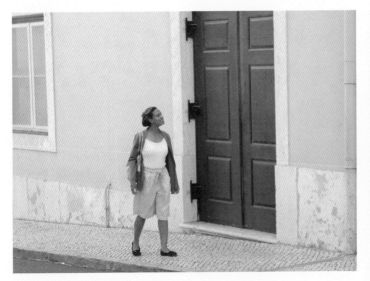

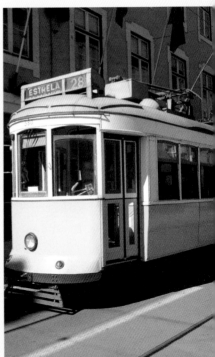

Exploring the ancient streets of Lisbon, Portugal.

At right: Here comes the bright yellow Remodelado Tram, Lisbon, Portugal.

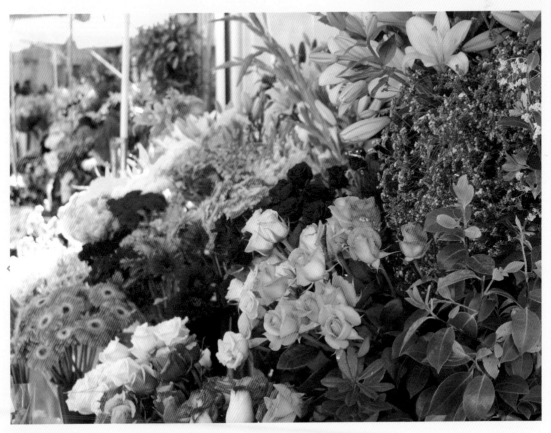

Sunday morning at the market in Lisbon, Portugal.

Lisbon sat tall and proud on the water. Her streets, narrow and inclined, held so many treasures.

I followed N'Djamena up Lisbon's narrow, cobblestoned streets. It was hot—late July. My 23-month-old was strapped to my chest in his carrier. His warm, fuzzy head bobbed from side to side as he slept, and a pool of sweat formed between his head and my cleavage. Irritated from the heat and craving a very large dish of gelato from the vantage point of a cool café, I sucked up my discomfort and quietly forged forward, following my sister's lead. Intent on shopping and free of the waterfalls of sweat that cascaded unfaltering down my face, she seemed oblivious to the heat as we popped in and out of boutiques, many of which weren't air-conditioned.

We'd been at it all morning; yet she was far from slowing down. My sister, stilettos tapping rhythmically on her swift feet, was almost galloping. I struggled to keep up with her despite being decked out in sensible "new mom" sneakers. With the growing weight of my son and the large backpack on my back that served as a diaper bag slowing me down, the best I could do was to keep a visual on N'Djamena's sleek chignon and listen for the click of her heels to keep up.

We became separated about 20 feet apart by a group of Italian tourists. N'Djamena paused to glance at her phone and then sprinted excitedly around a corner. Just like that, she was gone. I blinked, standing exhausted in a pool of sweat in the space where I last saw her. Nothing.

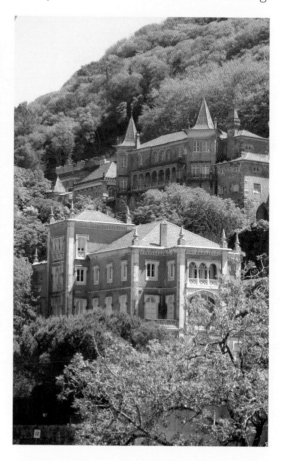

Flamenco dancer in Lisbon, Portugal.

At right: The storybook buildings in Sintra, Portugal.

Just as I was beginning to panic, I heard her excited squeal to the left.

"Look!" She waved me toward her. I rounded the corner to yet another narrow nondescript street sloping downward toward the water.

"There it is!" Her slender hand pointed toward an elegant brick building. The sign overhead read "Perfumaria."

Curiosity didn't even register; I was simply relieved a break was in sight. My gait matched hers as we made our way briskly inside. All I wanted was air-conditioning, and I hoped the shop wouldn't be overpowering in aroma and nauseating.

The scent of jasmine and bergamot cocooned me as I burst through the door. I stopped in my tracks, transfixed. Dimly lit candles flickered throughout the shop, revealing a collection of beautiful glass bottles filled with liquids of different colors and appeal. Along the far wall, large copper vats bubbled with distilled flower essences. Steam percolated inside bulbs of glass. There was a Siamese cat lounging nonchalantly beside a vase of plump ballet pink peonies.

N'Djamena winked at me before taking off toward a shelf of copper pots. So, this was a perfumaria? My irritation dissipated as my skin began to cool, my senses reinvigorated. I had been expecting a shop that sold perfume, similar to the annoying, brightly lit, duty-free shops in airports where you're offered inexpensive versions of expensive things you didn't want in the first place. This was not that experience. It was like stepping back in time. The shop

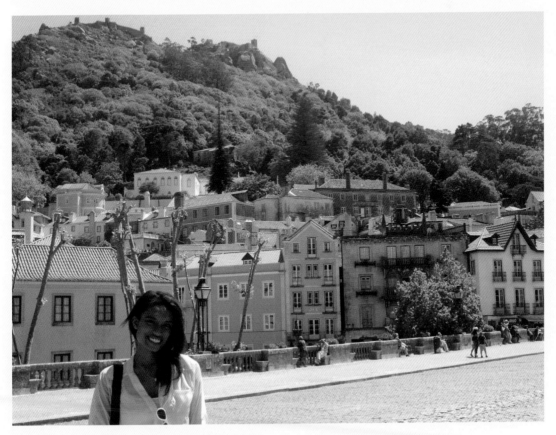

My sister, N'Djamena, in scenic Sintra, Portugal.

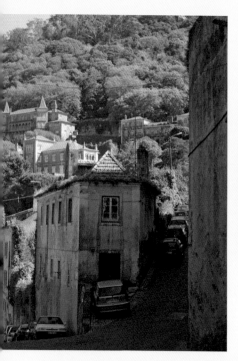

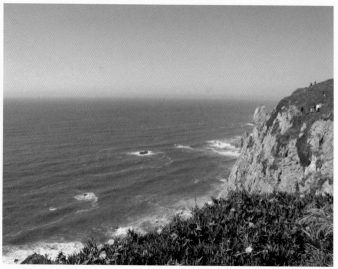

Cascais, Portugal, at the edge of the world.

At left: The steep and winding streets of old Sintra, Portugal.

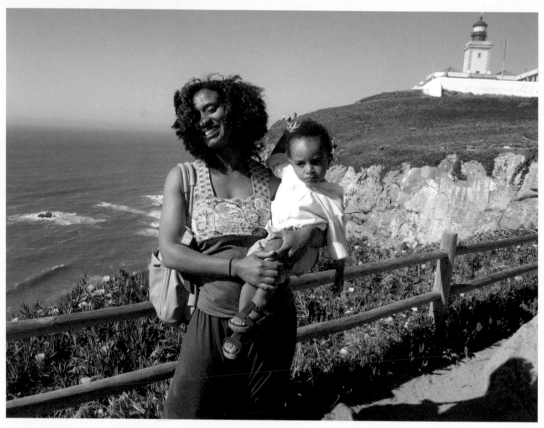

With my son, near a lighthouse in Cascais, Portugal.

had probably not been updated since the Victorian era, minus the air-conditioning. There was no plastic; the store was lit by gas lamps and candles, and the labels were all handwritten in perfect script. Pure floral extracts and essences waited to be sampled. There were floral oils and floral waters, perfume oils, and colognes.

N'Djamena and I, wide eyed, lingered from bottle to bottle, taking in the fragrances one by one. The woman behind the counter, who had lived in Massachusetts for some time, spoke perfect English and helped us mix and create our own blends. She briefed us about the history of floral waters and how they had arrived in Lisbon with the Moors, like the art and architecture, enhancing and adding to the indigenous culture and traditions.

The small perfumaria in Lisbon was the most extraordinary surprise find. I had stumbled into an ancient world of pure plant fragrances, each aroma taking me on a sensual journey to places old and new. I left with a bag full of floral waters and a mind buzzing with ideas for blending the waters into my handmade lotions and products.

We rode a graffiti-coated streetcar back to the hotel that night, relishing the city of Lisbon, a gorgeous blur of Islamic tile, ornate architecture, narrow cobblestone streets, and the unmistakably melancholy melody of Fado music.

Floral water is water that holds a floral aroma as well as the essence of the flower. Characteristics of floral water are similar to those of their essential oils. Floral waters are made in one of two ways. They're either steam distilled or blended. Steam-distilled floral waters are also known as hydrosol and are gathered in a similar way as essential oils are obtained through steam

distillation of water. When floral waters are steam distilled, they require a smaller quantity of botanicals-to-water ratio than with essential oil. Hydrosols are excellent for populations that may be sensitive to essential oils, with most hydrosols being safe for pregnant women and children.

Floral waters can also be created by mixing purified water with essential oils or by soaking blossoms in water as if making tea. These floral waters are great for toners, sprays, shampoos, and hair rinses. They can also be used in cooking and baking. You just want to make sure that the essential oil you're working with is food grade and/or ingestible. Though similar to a tea in which herbs are steeped in boiling water for consumption, herbal infusions are a bit more intense. Herbal infusions are steeped for at least four hours (and up to 10) and use a larger quantity of herbs-to-water ratio. Infusions provide many more times the amount of nutrition than tea. Water infusions are typically done to promote good health (for example, boosting immunity during cold season) and can

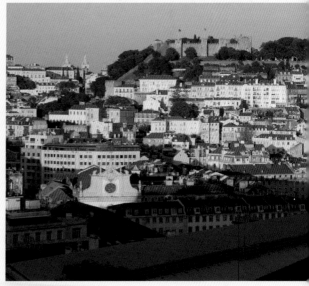

Beyond the palace walls in Cascais, Portugal.

be consumed medicinally or used in body care recipes that require water.

Oil herbal infusions are another way to create an infusion for body care. Using this method, dried flower and herbs are mixed with an oil of choice and steeped for several months. To prevent molding and bacteria, herbs must be fully dry before infusion in the oil. Infusions are created by filling half a jar of herb to the top with an oil. Set the jar in the sun for three months and shake daily. Strain, and then transfer to permanent storage containers.

There are so many different ways to use floral waters and herbal infusions in skin formulations. I'll outline some of my favorite recipes in the following pages.

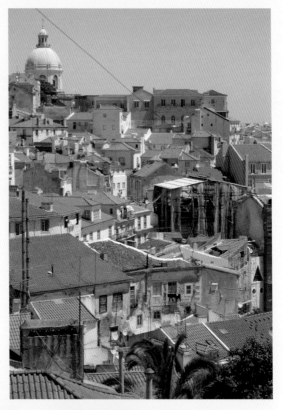

The red clay rooftops of Cascais, Portugal.

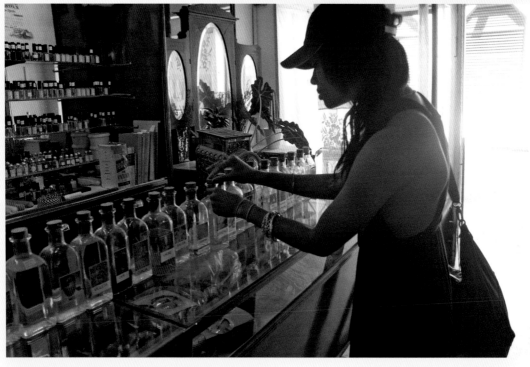

A visit to the perfumaria.

CALMING FACE MIST

This cooling mist is gentle enough for the most sensitive skin and powerful enough to pacify acne and other inflammatory conditions.

WHAT YOU'LL NEED:

- 2 cups purified water
- 1 cup fresh mint leaves
- ½ large cucumber, sliced
- 10 drops frankincense essential oil
- 5 drops rose absolute essential oil

WHAT TO DO:

1. Bring water to a boil in a large pot.
2. Add the mint leaves to the water once it has boiled and simmer on low heat for 15 minutes.
3. Add the cucumber slices and let the mint and cucumber steep for an hour, giving the water a chance to cool.
4. Strain the liquid from the pot using a cheesecloth. Repeat as many times as necessary to filter out any sediment.
5. Add the essential oils and shake to blend.

Yield:
One 8-ounce spray bottle

Preparation time:
75 minutes

Indications:
This is a light and calming gentle face mist.

Usage:
Spray 1–3 squirts on your face or neck to calm and soften skin.

Storage:
Store in the refrigerator for up to a month.

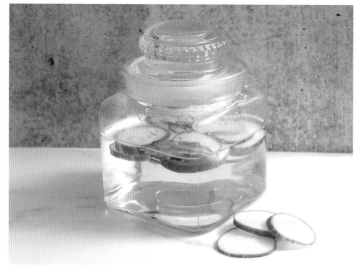

Calming Face Mist.

SKIN-BRIGHTENING MIST

Freshen and brighten dull, tired skin with this aromatic mist.

WHAT YOU'LL NEED:

- 1 large lemon
- 2 cups filtered water
- 2 tablespoons fresh lavender buds
- 1 cup fresh rose petals
- ½ cup fresh spearmint
- ¼ cup witch hazel
- 5 drops lavender essential oil
- 5 drops rose absolute essential oil

WHAT TO DO:

1. Rinse and slice the lemon.
2. Bring water to a boil in a pot.
3. Add to the boiling water the lemon, lavender, rose petals, and spearmint.
4. Reduce heat to a low simmer for 30 minutes.
5. Cover the mixture and cool for an hour, and then strain with a fine cheesecloth.
6. Add the witch hazel and essential oils and mix thoroughly.

Yield:
One 12-ounce spray bottle

Preparation time:
75 minutes

Indications:
Brighten and revitalize facial skin with this toner.

Usage:
Spray 1–3 squirts on a clean, dry face after washing.

Storage:
Store in the refrigerator for up to a month.

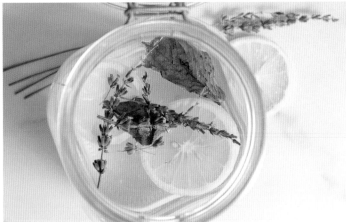

Skin-Brightening Mist.

MOOD-BOOSTING FRAGRANCE BODY MIST

Encourage feelings of joy, peace, and bliss with this beautifully aromatic body spray.

WHAT YOU'LL NEED:

- 5 ounces of 100 proof vodka
- *Essential oils:* Everyone will have a different preference when it comes to the strength of perfumes and sprays. The indicated number of drops below may be decreased or increased proportionally depending on whether the aroma is too strong or not strong enough. If a stronger aroma is preferred, up to 1½ ounces of your entire formulation may be essential oils. Anything more than 1½ ounces will not provide enough dilution and may irritate the skin.
  - ~ 50 drops cedarwood essential oil
  - ~ 50 drops ylang ylang essential oil
  - ~ 30 drops grapefruit essential oil
  - ~ 30 drops vetiver essential oil
- ½ tablespoon vegetable glycerin
- 4 tablespoons purified water

WHAT TO DO:

1. Blend the alcohol and essential oils together slowly.
2. In a separate container, mix the glycerin and water together.
3. Once both mixtures are uniform, combine the two together.
4. Let the liquid mixture set in a dark, cool place for 2 weeks. Shake each day to combine and settle the ingredients.

Yield:
One 8-ounce tinted glass spray bottle

Preparation time:
10 minutes (2-week wait before use)

Indications:
Floral, citrus, and earth notes combine in this blend that is both mood enhancing and grounding to promote a sense of balance and tranquility.

Usage:
Spritz onto yourself as a perfume as often as you like.

Storage:
Store in a cobalt or amber glass bottle away from direct sunlight for a year.

RELAXING FRAGRANCE BODY MIST

Relax and unwind with this tranquility-inducing body spray.

WHAT YOU'LL NEED:

- 5 ounces 100 proof vodka
- *Essential oils:* Everyone will have a different preference when it comes to the strength of perfumes and sprays. The indicated number of drops below may be decreased or increased proportionally depending on whether the aroma is too strong or not strong enough. If a stronger aroma is preferred, up to 1½ ounces of your entire formulation may be essential oils. Anything more than 1½ ounces will not provide enough dilution and may irritate the skin.
  - ~ 40 drops lavender essential oil
  - ~ 40 drops bergamot essential oil
  - ~ 25 drops jasmine essential oil
- ½ tablespoon vegetable glycerin
- 4 tablespoons purified water

Yield:
One 8-ounce spray bottle

Preparation time:
10 minutes (2-week wait time)

Indications:
This floral and calming body mist will encourage relaxation and calm.

Usage:
Spritz onto yourself as a perfume as often as you like.

Storage:
Store in a cobalt or amber glass bottle away from direct sunlight.

WHAT TO DO:

1. Blend the alcohol and essential oils together slowly.
2. In a separate container, mix the glycerin and water together.
3. Once both mixtures are uniform, combine the two together.
4. Let the liquid mixture set in a dark, cool place for 2 weeks. Shake each day to combine and settle the ingredients.

WOODSY/EARTHY PERFUME SPRAY

Inspired by a late autumn walk in the woods, this perfume spray is long lasting and gently grounding.

WHAT YOU'LL NEED:

- 5 ounces 100 proof vodka
- *Essential oils:* Everyone will have a different preference when it comes to the strength of perfumes and sprays. The indicated number of drops below may be decreased or increased proportionally depending on whether the aroma is too strong or not strong enough. If a stronger aroma is preferred, up to 1½ ounces of your entire formulation may be essential oils. Anything more than 1½ ounces will not provide enough dilution and may irritate the skin.
  - ~ 35 drops sandalwood essential oil
  - ~ 30 drops vetiver essential oil
  - ~ 15 drops patchouli essential oil
  - ~ 20 drops lime essential oil
- ½ tablespoon vegetable glycerin
- 1 ounce purified water

Yield:
One 8-ounce spray bottle

Preparation time:
10 minutes (2-week wait time)

Indications:
This woodsy and grounding perfume spray provides a light to medium long-lasting aroma.

Usage:
Spritz directly onto your skin as a perfume as often as needed.

Storage:
Store in an amber or cobalt glass container out of direct sunlight and heat.

WHAT TO DO:

1. Combine the alcohol and essential oils slowly.
2. In a separate container, blend the glycerin and water.
3. Combine the alcohol and essential oil mixture with the glycerin and water mixture.
4. Let the mixture rest for 2 weeks in a cool, dark place. Shake each day to combine and settle ingredients.

FLORAL PERFUME SPRAY

Inspired by a springtime ramble through a flower garden, the alluring floral notes in this perfume spray are grounded with a soothing citrus undertone.

WHAT YOU'LL NEED:

- 5 ounces 100 proof vodka
- *Essential oils:* Everyone will have a different preference when it comes to the strength of perfumes and sprays. The indicated number of drops below may be decreased or increased proportionally depending on whether the aroma is too strong or not strong enough. If a stronger aroma is preferred, up to 1½ ounces of your entire formulation may be essential oils. Anything more than 1½ ounces will not provide enough dilution and may irritate the skin.
  - ~ 40 drops rose absolute essential oil
  - ~ 30 drops ylang ylang essential oil
  - ~ 20 drops rose geranium essential oil
  - ~ 20 drops bergamot essential oil
- ½ tablespoon vegetable glycerin
- 1 ounce purified water

Yield:
One 8-ounce spray bottle

Preparation time:
10 minutes (2-week wait time)

Indications:
This complex floral perfume spray provides a light to medium long-lasting aroma.

Usage:
Spritz directly onto your skin as a perfume as often as needed.

Storage:
Store in an amber or cobalt glass container out of direct sunlight and heat.

WHAT TO DO:

1. Combine the alcohol and essential oils slowly.
2. In a separate container, blend the glycerin and water.
3. Combine the alcohol and essential oil mixture with the glycerin and water mixture.
4. Let the mixture rest for 2 weeks in a cool, dark place. Shake each day to combine and settle ingredients.

SPICY PERFUME SPRAY

The best of autumnal spices grounded with the earthy aroma of cedar, this is a gentle perfume spray, reminiscent of Grandma's kitchen during the holidays.

WHAT YOU'LL NEED:

- 5 ounces 100 proof vodka
- *Essential oils:* Everyone will have a different preference when it comes to the strength of perfumes and sprays. The indicated number of drops below may be decreased or increased proportionally depending on whether the aroma is too strong or not strong enough. If a stronger aroma is preferred, up to 1½ ounces of your entire formulation may be essential oils. Anything more than 1½ ounces will not provide enough dilution and may irritate the skin.
  - ~ 30 drops nutmeg essential oil
  - ~ 25 drops cedarwood essential oil
  - ~ 30 drops clove essential oil
  - ~ 20 drops vanilla essential oil
- ½ tablespoon vegetable glycerin
- 1 ounce purified water

Yield:
One 8-ounce spray bottle

Preparation time:
10 minutes (2-week wait time)

Indications:
This spicy, autumn-inspired perfume spray provides a light to medium long-lasting aroma.

Usage:
Spritz directly onto your skin as a perfume as often as needed.

Storage:
Store in an amber or cobalt glass container out of direct sunlight and heat.

WHAT TO DO:

1. Combine the alcohol and essential oils slowly.
2. In a separate container, blend the glycerin and water.
3. Combine the alcohol and essential oil mixture with the glycerin and water mixture.
4. Let the mixture rest for 2 weeks in a cool dark place. Shake each day to combine and settle ingredients.

CITRUS/HERB PERFUME SPRAY

Imagine summertime in Tuscany, a complex hint of citrus combined with wild herbs. If the summer sun had an aroma, this would be it.

WHAT YOU'LL NEED:

- 5 ounces 100 proof vodka
- *Essential oils:* Everyone will have a different preference when it comes to the strength of perfumes and sprays. The indicated number of drops below may be decreased or increased proportionally depending on whether the aroma is too strong or not strong enough. If a stronger aroma is preferred, up to 1½ ounces of your entire formulation may be essential oils. Anything more than 1½ ounces will not provide enough dilution and may irritate the skin.
  - 40 drops bergamot essential oil
  - 25 drops lemon essential oil
  - 15 drops thyme essential oil
- ½ tablespoon vegetable glycerin
- 1 ounce purified water

Yield:
One 8-ounce spray bottle

Preparation time:
10 minutes (2-week wait time)

Indications:
This light, uplifting perfume spray provides a light to medium long-lasting aroma.

Usage:
Spritz directly onto your skin as a perfume as often as needed.

Storage:
Store in an amber or cobalt glass container out of direct sunlight and heat.

WHAT TO DO:

1. Combine the alcohol and essential oils slowly.
2. In a separate container, blend glycerin and water.
3. Combine the alcohol and essential oil mixture with the glycerin and water mixture.
4. Let the mixture rest for 2 weeks in a cool, dark place. Shake each day to combine and settle ingredients.

COOLING SUMMER FACE MIST

This may be the most blissful thing to return home to after a long day out and about in the humid heat of the summer. Store in the refrigerator and spritz on your face and neck to cool skin and gently draw out dirt and grime. This works wonders after a beach day!

WHAT YOU'LL NEED:

- 2 ounces rosewater
- 1 ounce aloe vera juice
- 1 ounce witch hazel
- 20 drops lavender essential oil

WHAT TO DO:

1. Measure ingredients and add directly to a sterile spray bottle.
2. Shake to mix.

Yield:
4 ounces

Preparation time:
5 minutes

Indications:
This skin-pacifying spray is a wonderful treat after being outside in the summer sun. It also works wonders to soothe sunburn.

Usage:
Spritz on your face and neck to combat a steamy summer day.

Storage:
Store in the refrigerator for up to a month. Step outside, go for a run, take a walk, go to work—then, when you come back home, go straight to your refrigerator (don't forget and let it disappear behind the leftovers), shake your spray bottle, and mist away!

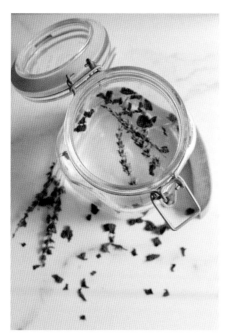

Cooling Summer Face Mist.

FLORAL FACIAL TONER

Clarify skin, unclog pores, and reduce inflammation with this aromatic, hormone-balancing facial toner. It's gentle enough for sensitive skin, effective for acne-prone skin, and supportive of mature skin.

WHAT YOU'LL NEED:

- 1 ounce rosewater
- 1 ounce witch hazel
- 5 drops lavender essential oil
- 3 drops ylang ylang essential oil

WHAT TO DO:

1. Combine the rosewater and witch hazel in a (preferably glass) spray pump container.
2. Measure and drop the essential oils into the bottle.
3. Shake container to mix ingredients.

Yield:
2 ounces

Preparation time:
5 minutes

Indications:
Cleansing, clarifying, and moisturizing, this toner works well for combination, mature, and inflamed skin.

Usage:
Spritz 1–3 pumps on a clean, dry face.

Storage:
Store in a cool, dry place for up to 6 months.

Southern Africa and Western Europe, 2007

I can still feel the sun on my face and the wind in my hair, but what I remember most is the vivid red color of the clay road. I had never seen that hue of red before—terra cotta, really. We were in Swaziland, my best friend and housemate Tamika and I, on our first vacation after six months of teaching in southeastern Mozambique. Eager to take in new sights and experiences, but on a tight budget, we planned the cheapest weeklong getaway that we could find: a no-frills escape across the western border into Swaziland.

After traveling from Inhambane, Mozambique, to Maputo, Mozambique (the capital city, near the Swazi border), in a rickety cargo van with patches of floor missing, we transferred to an even more fragile and dilapidated frame of a bus that jostled us over gaping potholed streets into Mbabane, Swaziland. Swaziland had a different energy entirely. Back in the English-speaking world, Swaziland seemed formal and slightly sterile. The buildings, boxy and low, reminded me of California. Mbabane, our host city, was a clean, tidy city with a white stucco Anglican church on every corner. It was also a very hilly city, which made our prospect of getting around by foot tricky, especially since we were wearing flip-flops and pulling rolling suitcases. Having had enough of cargo vans for the time being, we decided to try our luck at hitchhiking the rest of the way and were fortunate enough to catch a ride in the back of a pickup truck. Hitchhiking in southern Africa was a very common practice, one that we had come to rely on to get from place to place.

It was the perfect overcast day. The sun, respectful of our skin and eyes, kept her distance behind clouds. We smoothly rolled over the soft red earth, eyes wide

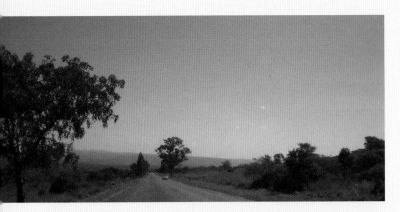

The long road to Mbabane, Swaziland.

Below: Bulls at pasture in the Swaziland countryside.

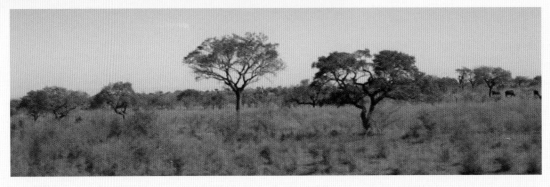

as we took in the landscape around us. Hungry-looking cows grazed the vibrant foliage, their ribs protruding despite the bounty before them. I leaned back against the side of the truck, bracing myself with my arms. Above me, the sky hung heavy with cloudy gray dew; below, the earth lay before us, red and moist. Somewhere between sky and earth I sat, perfectly content.

"It's so red," Tamika commented, nodding toward the road.

And it was. I'd never before seen earth that looked so rich and otherworldly. It had rained the day before, and the soil, still moist, reminded me of the clay I used to play with in elementary school—my teacher's "special clay" that needed to be oven dried, which we'd been allowed to tinker with when we were behaving well. Proudly I'd shuffle my creations home, where they'd be displayed on the windowsill in the living room.

"Is that clay?" I wondered aloud, jogged by memory.

"I think so." Tamika shrugged.

An hour later, we arrived at our destination. We jumped from the bed of the truck, our Havaianas sinking into the squishy clay earth beneath the weight of our camping backpacks. It was a long and slippery trek, uphill. My toes dug into my flip-flops as the red clay earth rose over the edges of my shoes and settled into the spaces between my toes. By the time we made it to our hostel, our ankles were caked in mud. Every step sent our heels sliding over the sides of our shoes. Once settled in our tiny, dim room, we took turns showering to wipe the clay earth from our feet and then hand washed our shoes. The mud had managed to get everywhere.

I remembered my Swaziland adventure a year later when I was in Montmartre, France, where I lay, face up in a reclining chair, with an aesthetician, an enormous light attached to her head, slathering my face in a mask of cold green clay that looked more gray than green. Shocked at first by its coolness, I felt the clay begin to settle on my face, a comforting, moist weight. I closed my eyes as she massaged my cheekbones and décolleté with her knuckles. It was my first clay facial, and as I lay in the heated chair, eyes closed and a smile on my lips, I wondered whether the women who I'd seen in some of the far-flung villages in Swaziland and Mozambique, whose skin appeared reddened, used the clay earth to heal and energize their bodies as well.

At the end of my facial, when all of the clay had been wiped clean, my skin felt alive and light. When I made it back home to New York, after my summer vacation in France, I was obsessed with clay. After a bit of research at home, I began to experiment with making clay masks and then clay powders. Before I knew it,

I had makeup, toothpaste, deodorant, dry shampoo, body powder, and face and hair masks.

Clays, which are known to draw out toxins and impurities, have been used in Europe throughout history to treat a plethora of skin problems and digestive disorders. My research also revealed that my instincts about the women in southern Africa were correct. Red clay had been used as a mask among the Himba people in the form of Otjize, a mixture of mineral-rich clay, butterfat, and resin. As a mask, Otjize dries and then flakes off, revealing exfoliated smooth skin. While intact in the form of a mask, the Otjize protects skin, scalp, and hair from the sun while providing hydration.

There are as many different uses for clays as there are types. In a modern context, clay is often used cosmetically to draw impurities out of the skin and provide gentle exfoliation. Red, green, gray, brown,

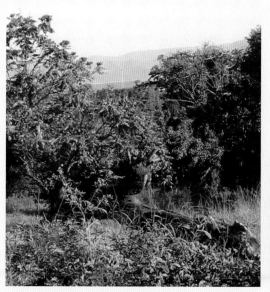

The flora of Mbabane, Swaziland.

Below: The view from Mbabane, Swaziland.

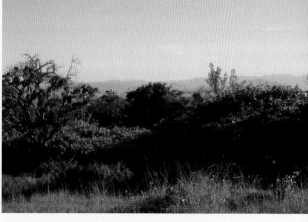

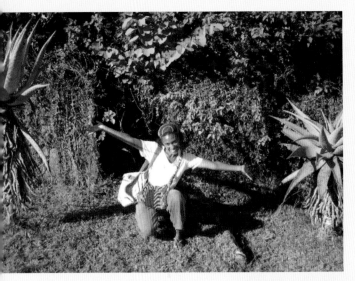

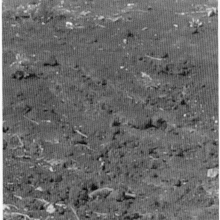

Red earth.

Fresh off the bus and exploring Mbabane, Swaziland, by foot.

At right: Cows on the side of the road in the Swaziland countryside.

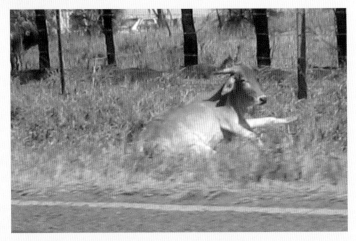

Below: School's out! Children at play in the pickup line, Mbabane, Swaziland.

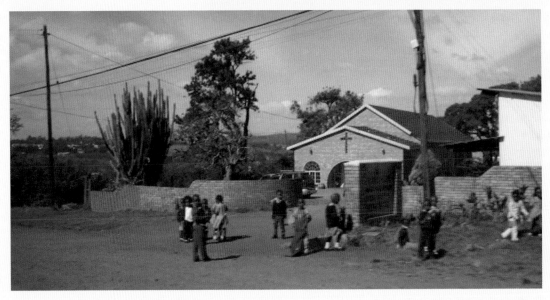

and charcoal clays have been restoring balance both internally and externally for thousands of years. Typically and most familiarly used in the form of a mask, clay can also be used as an exfoliating agent, as a topical powder for absorbing oils on the skin, or as a deodorant base for neutralizing odors. The chart below identifies the benefits of some of the most common cosmetic clays in use today:

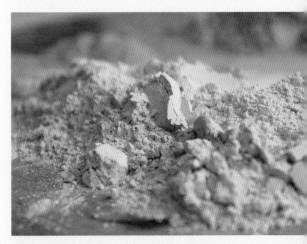

Clay powder.

Moroccan Red Clay
Excellent for both skin and hair, Moroccan red clay is gentle enough for sensitive skin and effectively draws impurities from skin and scalp.

≈ Absorbs oil
≈ Evens skin tone
≈ Reduces acne
≈ Increases skin elasticity

White Kaolin Clay
White kaolin clay is extremely fine and soft and is one of the gentlest clays, making it compatible with the most sensitive skin.

≈ Unclogs pores
≈ Exfoliates skin
≈ Stimulates circulation
≈ Doesn't dry the skin out, making it ideal for sensitive skin
≈ Detoxifies skin

French Green Clay
French green clay is healing and promotes detoxification due to its extreme effectiveness at drawing out oils and impurities.

≈ Anti-inflammatory
≈ Detoxifies
≈ Natural deodorant
≈ Calms irritated skin
≈ Absorbs oil

Bentonite Clay
Bentonite clay is highly absorbent and is effective at absorbing toxins. Full of minerals and composed of volcanic ash, bentonite is both alkaline and nutrient rich.

≈ Absorbs oil
≈ Tightens skin
≈ Brightens skin
≈ Reduces the appearance of scars
≈ Exfoliates skin
≈ Softens skin
≈ Boosts immunity

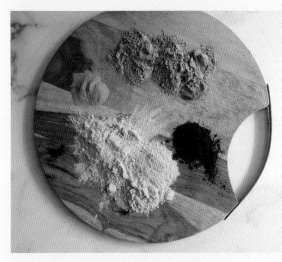

Assortment of clay powders.

From face masks to toothpastes, scalp treatments and deodorant, there are so many different ways to use clay in bath and beauty formulations. I'll outline some of my favorite recipes in the following pages.

SOOTHING CHARCOAL MASK

Draw dirt, bacteria, and toxins from your skin while controlling oil secretions with this powerful, detoxifying facial mask.

WHAT YOU'LL NEED:

- 1 teaspoon bentonite clay
- 1 teaspoon activated charcoal
- 1 teaspoon rosewater
- 1 teaspoon full-fat plain yogurt
- 3 drops tea tree essential oil

WHAT TO DO:

Do not use aluminum spoons, whisks, or bowls for this recipe, as aluminum will deactivate the bentonite clay.

1. Combine the bentonite clay with the activated charcoal, mixing with a spoon until uniform.
2. In a separate dish, combine the rosewater, yogurt, and tea tree essential oil.
3. Add the clay and charcoal mixture to the yogurt, rosewater, and tea tree mixture.

Yield:
Single-use batch that can fit into a 1-ounce container

Preparation time:
10 minutes

Indications:
This antimicrobial mask detoxifies, deep cleans pores, tones skin, and calms acne.

Usage:
Apply to a clean face. Leave on for 10–15 minutes until dry, and then rinse.

Storage:
Store in the refrigerator for up to a month.

CHARCOAL AND HONEY EXFOLIATING MASK

Support deep and gentle exfoliation with this detoxifying and moisturizing facial mask.

WHAT YOU'LL NEED:

- 1 teaspoon bentonite clay
- 1 teaspoon activated charcoal
- ½ teaspoon apple cider vinegar
- 1 teaspoon raw honey
- 3 drops tea tree essential oil

WHAT TO DO:

Do not use aluminum spoons, whisks, or bowls for this recipe, as aluminum will deactivate the bentonite clay.

1. Combine the bentonite clay and activated charcoal in a bowl until uniform.
2. In a separate container, mix the apple cider vinegar, raw honey, and essential oil.
3. Add the bentonite clay and activated charcoal mixture to the apple cider vinegar, raw honey, and essential oil mixture.

Yield:
Single-serving mask that can fit in about a ½-ounce container

Preparation time:
10 minutes

Indications:
This detoxifying mask absorbs impurities, calms skin, draws out heavy metals and toxins, regenerates skin tissue, and prevents and removes blackheads.

Usage:
Apply to a clean face. Leave on for 10–15 minutes until dry, and then rinse.

Storage:
Store in the refrigerator for up to a month.

MOISTURIZING AND CURL-ENHANCING MOROCCAN RED CLAY HAIR MASK

Deep condition, reduce frizz, and seal moisture into your hair shaft with this soothing hair mask.

WHAT YOU'LL NEED:

- 1 tablespoon coconut oil (softened)
- 1 tablespoon Jamaican black castor oil
- 4 tablespoons water
- 4 tablespoons apple cider vinegar
- ½ cup Moroccan red clay

WHAT TO DO:

1. If your coconut oil is hard, soften it by running the jar under warm water.
2. Combine softened coconut oil and Jamaican black castor oil in a bowl.
3. In a separate container, combine water and apple cider vinegar.
4. Add the red clay to the water and apple cider vinegar mixture. Combine until smooth.
5. Add the red clay mixture to the coconut and castor oil mixture. Mix until smooth and uniform.

Yield:
One 10-ounce jar

Preparation time:
15 minutes

Indications:
This mask with anti-inflammatory and antiseptic properties soothes the scalp, cleans hair without depleting natural oils, stimulates new hair growth, and leaves hair shiny and lustrous.

Usage:
Apply generously to hair and scalp. Wear a plastic shower cap and leave in hair for at least 1 hour but up to 6 hours before rinsing in the shower.

Storage:
Store in a cool, dry place for up to 6 weeks.

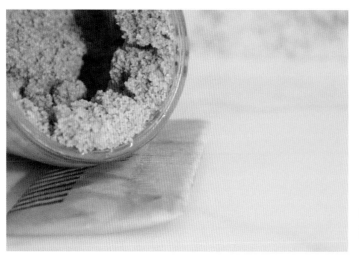

Moisturizing and Curl-Enhancing Moroccan Red Clay Hair Mask.

TOOTHPASTE WITH WHITE KAOLIN CLAY

Clean and whiten teeth with this refreshing, remineralizing toothpaste.

WHAT YOU'LL NEED:

- 1 teaspoon baking soda
- 1 teaspoon coconut oil
- 5 drops tea tree essential oil
- 10 drops peppermint essential oil
- 3 drops clove essential oil
- 1 teaspoon xylitol
- ¼ cup white kaolin clay
- 2 tablespoons purified mineral water

WHAT TO DO:

1. In a bowl, combine the baking soda and softened coconut oil. If your coconut oil is hard, soften it by running the jar under warm water.
2. Add the essential oil and xylitol and continue mixing until smooth.
3. Add clay and water and continue mixing until uniform and almost whipped in texture.

Yield:
One 2-ounce jar/container

Preparation time:
10 minutes

Indications:
Great for sensitive teeth, this toothpaste remineralizes teeth, creates a healthy pH for the mouth, and whitens teeth.

Usage:
Put a pea-sized amount on your toothbrush and rinse fully when finished brushing. Use twice a day.

Storage:
Store in the refrigerator for up to a month.

COOLING SPRING/SUMMER GREEN CLAY MASK

Slough away tired, dry, winter skin with this revitalizing mask. Gentle and moisturizing, this mask is ideal for sensitive, acne-prone, and mature skin.

WHAT YOU'LL NEED:

- 1 tablespoon French green clay powder
- 1 tablespoon full-fat, plain Greek yogurt
- 1 tablespoon coconut oil (softened to room temperature)
- 1 tablespoon rosewater
- 1 teaspoon vegetable glycerin
- 5 drops rose essential oil

WHAT TO DO:

1. In a small bowl or dish, measure out your green clay powder and yogurt.
2. Mix with a spoon until smooth, and then add the softened coconut oil.
3. Mix until smooth, and then add the rosewater, vegetable glycerin, and essential oil.
4. Mix to a uniform paste-like consistency.

Yield:
2 ounces

Preparation time:
10 minutes

Indications:
This mask with antibacterial properties clears impurities from within pores, helps remove dead skin cells, combats dirt and pollution buildup, and softens, cleanses, and exfoliates skin.

Usage:
Apply liberally to face and neck. Leave on for 10 minutes before rinsing.

Storage:
Store in the refrigerator for up to a month.

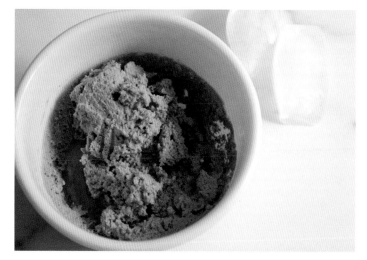

Cooling Spring/Summer Green Clay Mask.

BENTONITE CLAY CLEANSER

Deeply detoxify and control oil production with this powerful mask. Ideal for oily and combination skin, it also draws out impurities. Whiteheads and blackheads won't stand a chance.

WHAT YOU'LL NEED:

- 2 ounces bentonite clay
- 4 ounces organic unrefined coconut oil
- 20 drops of lavender essential oil

WHAT TO DO:

Do not use aluminum spoons, whisks, or bowls for this recipe, as aluminum will deactivate the bentonite clay.

1. Fill a jar with bentonite clay.
2. Top the jar off with coconut oil.
3. Add 2–5 drops of lavender essential oil per ounce.
4. Using a wooden or plastic spoon, mix everything together.
5. If you're working with a plastic top, shake the contents for even blending.
6. Make sure to gather the clay from the bottom of the jar.
7. If the coconut oil was melted to a liquid, refrigerate for 5 minutes; then stir and repeat until the coconut oil cleanser is creamy.

Yield:
6 ounces

Preparation time:
15 minutes

Indications:
This moisturizing and detoxifying cleanser with antimicrobial properties soothes acne, reduces inflammation, and draws out impurities.

Usage:
Apply to a clean face. Leave on for 15–20 minutes, and then rinse off.

Storage:
Store in a cool, dry place out of direct sunlight for up to 2 weeks.

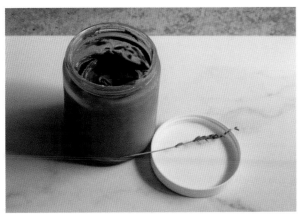

Bentonite Clay Cleanser.

LAVENDER DEODORANT POWDER

Fragrant and effective, this lavender deodorant powder is extremely easy to apply to underarms, feet, and anywhere else you may need a little deodorizing. It's great for babies, too. In fact, I may need to make another batch for my little one because I'm having so much fun using this silky lavender-scented powder. This is perfect if you need to go outside on a humid, sticky day.

WHAT YOU'LL NEED:

- 4 ounces cornstarch
- 2 ounces French green clay
- 20 drops lavender essential oil

WHAT TO DO:

1. In a jar, combine cornstarch and French green clay.
2. Combine until uniformly blended (I screw on the cap and give the jar a good shake).
3. Tap the lid to make sure that the powder has fallen into the jar; then unscrew and add the lavender essential oil.
4. Screw the top on again and give the powder a good shake. Tap the lid again to encourage the powder to fall into the jar, and then open the lid.
5. Leave the lid off for an hour so that the powder can dry. Make sure the room is dry and not humid, or you won't have great results.
6. While the top is off the jar, take a hammer and nail and punch holes (a small circle in the center of the lid with holes close together is best) so the powder can flow freely when needed.

Yield:
6 ounces

Preparation time:
75 minutes

Indications:
This gentle and nonirritating powder with antibacterial and antimicrobial properties reduces odor, softens skin, and draws out toxins.

Usage:
With your fingertips or using a powder poof, apply directly to the underarms as often as needed. Note: This is not an antiperspirant.

Storage:
Store in a cool, dry place for up to a year.

GREEN CLAY FACE MASK

Fight inflammation, calm acne, remove toxins, and restore moisture and pH balance to your skin with this green clay mask.

WHAT YOU'LL NEED:

- 1 tablespoon green clay powder
- ¼ teaspoon turmeric powder
- 1 teaspoon grapeseed oil
- Plain full-fat yogurt or rosewater

WHAT TO DO:

1. In a bowl, mix the green clay powder and turmeric together until blended.
2. Add the grapeseed oil followed by the yogurt or rosewater (enough to create a paste-like texture).

Yield:
1 ounce

Preparation time:
10 minutes

Indications:
This mask with antiseptic, anti-bacterial, and anti-inflammatory properties detoxifies, calms, and conditions skin; draws out impurities; and reduces red-ness, acne, and rosacea.

Usage:
Apply to a clean, dry face and leave on for 10–15 minutes before rinsing. Once dry, rinse with warm water and pat your face dry with a towel.

Storage:
Store in the refrigerator for up to a month.

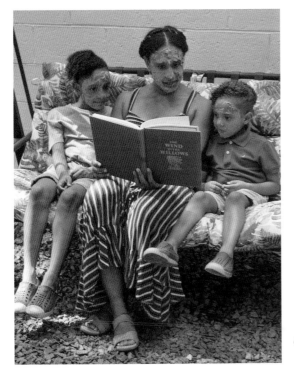

Green Clay Face Mask: Reading break!

OIL-ABSORBING TRANSLUCENT FACIAL POWDER

Use a powder puff or brush to set your makeup or apply to a clean face to help with oil absorption throughout the day. This silky, translucent facial powder is detoxifying and smells like a warm mug of hot chocolate.

WHAT YOU'LL NEED:

- ⊘ 2 teaspoons bentonite clay
- ⊘ 2 teaspoons cornstarch
- ⊘ 1 teaspoon cocoa powder*
- ⊘ ⅛ teaspoon turmeric*

* Add more or less cocoa powder and turmeric depending on skin tone.

WHAT TO DO:

1. You can prepare this blend directly in the storage jar. You'll want a container without a metal lid.
2. Combine the bentonite clay, cornstarch, cocoa powder, and turmeric. The quickest and most thorough way to do this is to screw on the top and shake vigorously.

Yield:
1 ounce

Preparation time:
5 minutes

Indications:
This oil-absorbing powder with anti-inflammatory properties creates a dewy glow, evens skin tone, and calms skin.

Usage:
Apply a light brushing to a clean, dry face using a makeup brush or powder pad on top of a favorite moisturizer or to set makeup.

Storage:
Store in a clean, dry place for up to 6 months.

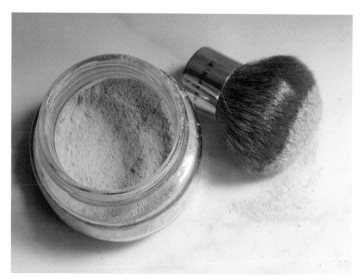

Oil-Absorbing Translucent Facial Powder.

COCONUT OIL AND GREEN CLAY FACIAL CLEANSER

Gently cleanse and exfoliate with this no-foam moisturizing cleanser. Tingly and refreshing, this facial cleanser works wonders on acne-prone and inflamed skin.

WHAT YOU'LL NEED:

- 1 tablespoon French green clay powder
- 1 tablespoon coconut oil
- 10 drops tea tree essential oil
- 1 teaspoon vegetable glycerin
- ¼ teaspoon vitamin E oil

WHAT TO DO:

1. In a container of choice (I always recommend glass because plastic can leach toxins into your product), mix the French green clay and coconut oil to an almost toothpaste-like consistency.
2. Add your tea tree, vegetable glycerin, and vitamin E oil and stir with a spoon until smooth.

Yield:
1 ounce

Preparation time:
10 minutes

Indications:
This cleanser is a mild exfoliant.

Usage:
Rub a dime-sized amount of cleanser onto moist skin in a circular motion, avoiding eyes. Rinse with warm water and pat face dry. Toner is an ideal next step.

Storage:
This will last 3 months easily, but because the batch size is relatively small, you'll probably need to make this every month.

ESSENTIAL OILS
NEW YORK CITY

Northeastern United States of America, 2003

I remember exactly where I was when I was first exposed to essential oils. It was 2003, I was a volunteer at the New York Open Center, and I had been scheduled to assist in an aromatherapy workshop. This was toward the beginning of my holistic studies, and I was open to learning and experiencing any and everything. I had heard of aromatherapy before and had a vague understanding of what it was, based mostly on the massages I'd had in which the masseuses had used aromatherapy oils. Those oils, combined with a massage, were like magic, transforming this tense New Yorker into a relaxed and joyful human. I was excited to learn more and experience aromatherapy independent of bodywork.

The New York Open Center was one of my first holistic "homes," and the best part of volunteering at the center was that I was able to sit in on and participate in the workshops and courses free of charge. It was a perfect arrangement for my public school teacher's budget. I came, I listened, I took notes, and I absorbed as much information as I could. I learned about master cleanses and liver detoxification. I learned about spirt animals and Native American flute meditations. I did vision boards and dream maps, and now I was ready and open to learn about aromatherapy.

For this particular workshop, the instructor passed around cotton balls and ziplock baggies. The first essential oil to be dropped on my cotton ball was lavender. The activity was to smell the cotton ball and record how the oil made us feel and/or any memories associated with the oil. Afterward, we would share as the

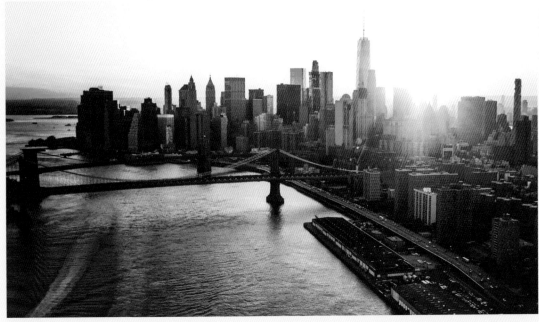
Franckreporter/E+ via Getty Images.

Manhattan skyline.

workshop leader discussed the properties of and uses of each oil. Each cotton ball was stored and saved in a baggie for future enjoyment.

We interacted with lavender, and I was reminded of my grandmother's house in Maryland during the summertime. Bergamot brought me back to making Italian sodas at the coffee shop where I had worked as a barista during college. Lemon reminded me of my kitchen in the morning during the seasonal transition from winter to spring. Peppermint took me back to snow days as a child growing up in Rochester, New York, and playing all day in shoulder-deep snow. Tea tree reminded me of an apothecary shop, eucalyptus stirred memories of cough drops, and sandalwood took me back to the fresh wood smell of my grandfather's carpentry shop. So many memories and emotions were contained in just one micro drop of essential oil. The workshop couldn't have been more than two hours. I can't even recall the name of the presenter, but a

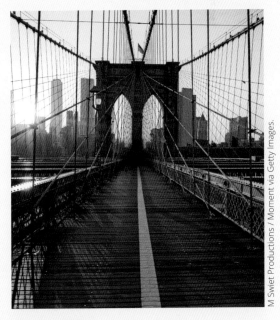
M Swiet Productions / Moment via Getty Images.

Brooklyn Bridge.

light had been turned on. I felt calm, invigorated, and dreamy all at the same time. I was hooked.

After the workshop, I walked uptown to the West Village. This was before the days when there was a Whole Foods in every New York City neighborhood with a carefully curated essential oil experience waiting for you in aisle 12. Instead, I spent the evening wandering from one tiny health food store to the next, crossing from the West to the East Village in search of essential oils to try. My collection really took off when my friend Elisha introduced me to the Mountain Rose Herbal website.

I enrolled in an aromatherapy certification course. There was so much that I wanted to learn and get from my experience with essential oils: I wanted to make perfumes. I wanted to make salves and ointments. I enjoyed creating a scent story for my apartment. I wanted to treat minor ailments and craft deliciously scented body lotions and oils.

Essential oils are natural chemical constituents derived directly from the stem, root, leaves, bark, seeds, resin, or petals of plants. Essential oils are extremely concentrated and can be used medicinally and for aromatherapy.

There are many fragrance oils out there composed of synthetic ingredients; therefore, when choosing fragrance and essences for your cosmetic blends, it's important to make sure that you're using pure essential oils. Pure essential oils, like many other things, can vary greatly when it comes to quality. The quality of an essential oil can be influenced by a multitude of factors, including how and where the plant is grown, the time of year and way the plant is harvested, where and how long the extraction of the essential oils takes place, the method of extraction used, and how the oil is bottled and stored.

Most essential oils are steam distilled. Steam distillation is the process of drawing oils out of plants with steam. Since water and essential oils (think water and oil) do not mix, the two compounds separate, and the essential oil is collected. Essential oils can also be extracted through cold-press extraction. When this happens, oils

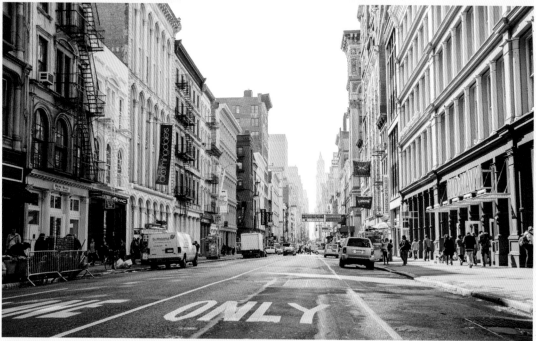

Soho, New York City.

are pressed out of the plant. This result is most common with citrus oils, in which the oil is pressed out of the peel, rind, and zest of the citrus fruit.

There are hundreds of essential oil options, but the following pages list some of my favorite oils to use for bath and beauty preparations.

Essential oil in cobalt container.

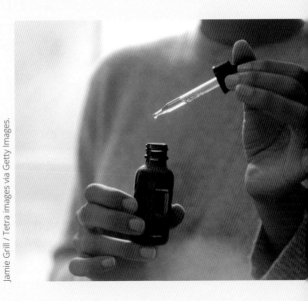

Jamie Grill / Tetra images via Getty Images.

ESSENTIAL OIL TYPES

ANGELICA ESSENTIAL OIL (*Angelica archangelica*)
This oil gives an earthy and herbaceous aroma.

Extraction process:	Steam distilled from the root
Geographic location of the plant:	France
Essential oil properties:	Carminative; circulation stimulant
Uses:	Combats stress, anxiety, and tension; builds strength and stamina; moisturizes; relieves indigestion and gas
Body care preparation suggestions:	Soaps, moisturizers, salves

BASIL ESSENTIAL OIL (*Ocimum basilicum*)
This oil gives a warm, herbaceous, and crisp aroma.

Extraction process:	Steam distilled from basil leaves
Geographic location of the plant:	Mediterranean and Asia
Essential oil properties:	Antibacterial, antifungal, heating
Uses:	Boosts mental clarity and alertness; promotes circulation
Body care preparation suggestions:	Soaps, salves

BERGAMOT ESSENTIAL OIL (*Citrus bergamia*)
This oil gives a spicy, citrusy, and tart aroma.

Extraction process:	Cold pressed from the citrus peel
Geographic location of the plant:	Italy and France
Essential oil properties:	Antidepressant and antiviral; hormone regulator
Uses:	Earl Grey tea; used by British to treat yellow fever
Body care preparation suggestions:	Perfumes, creams, lotions, deodorants

CEDARWOOD ESSENTIAL OIL (*Cedrus atlantica (Endl.) Manetti*)
This oil gives a woody, sweet, and warm aroma.

Extraction process:	Steam distilled from cedarwood
Geographic location of the plant:	Himalayas, Mediterranean region
Essential oil properties:	Expectorant, insect repellent, anti-anxiety, sedative
Uses:	Ceremonial/purification; used by Tibetans as incense in temples; heals skin infections; clears acne; tightens pores; reduces blemishes; balances oily skin
Body care preparation suggestions:	Perfumes, lotions, creams

CHAMOMILE (*Matricaria chamomilla*)
This oil gives a fruity, herbaceous, and sweet aroma.

Extraction process:	Steam distilled from the flowers of the chamomile plant
Geographic location of the plant:	Western Europe, Western Asia, India
Essential oil properties:	Inflammation reducer, sedative, calming
Uses:	Aids sleep; helps to heal wounds; moisturizes skin and hair
Body care preparation suggestions:	Salves, lotions, creams, hair conditioners

CINNAMON BARK ESSENTIAL OIL (*Cinnamomum cassia*)

This oil gives a spicy, earthy, and sweet aroma.

Extraction process:	Steam distilled from cinnamon bark
Geographic location of the plant:	Sri Lanka, China, Vietnam, Myanmar
Essential oil properties:	Antiviral, warm, grounding, analgesic, aphrodisiac
Uses:	Increases circulation; relieves pain; enhances libido
Body care preparation suggestions:	Perfumes, cosmetics, soaps, lotions, salves

CITRONELLA ESSENTIAL OIL (*Cymbopogon citronellol*)

This oil gives a floral, grassy, and citrusy aroma.

Extraction process:	Steam distilled from the leaves and stems of lemongrass
Geographic location of the plant:	Asia
Essential oil properties:	Nervine, antifungal, antibacterial
Uses:	Repels insects; treats lice in hair
Body care preparation suggestions:	Lotions, soaps, perfumes

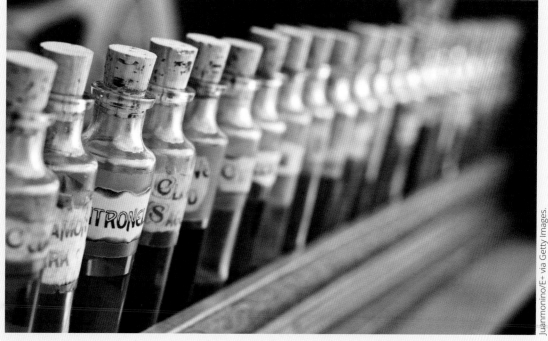

Essential oils.

Juanmonino/E+ via Getty Images.

CLARY SAGE ESSENTIAL OIL (*Salvia sclarea*)
This oil gives a dry, astringent, and slightly nutty aroma.

Extraction process:	Steam distilled from the sage herb
Geographic location of the plant:	Mediterranean, North Africa, Central Asia
Essential oil properties:	Mood booster, anti-anxiety, calming
Uses:	Affects the mood and creates a sense of calm; relieves anxiety and stress; helps with insomnia; helps with hormonal balance; relieves menstrual cramps; improves scalp health; stimulates hair growth; fights inflammation; treats depression and Alzheimer's disease; treats high blood pressure; treats periodontitis
Body care preparation suggestions:	Lotions, soaps, salves

CLOVE ESSENTIAL OIL (*Syzygium aromaticum*)
This oil gives a strong, spicy, and slightly earthy aroma.

Extraction process:	Steam distilled from the bud of the clove flower
Geographic location of the plant:	China
Essential oil properties:	Analgesic (pain relief), antibacterial, antimicrobial
Uses:	Historical: recorded in beauty formulations dating back to ancient China (226 BCE, when the emperor made his guests hold cloves in their mouths when speaking to ensure a pleasant and fragrant odor)
Body care preparation suggestions:	Mouthwash, soaps, toothpaste, salves, perfumes

COPAIBA ESSENTIAL OIL (*Copaifera*)
This oil gives a woody, sweet, and earthy aroma.

Extraction process:	Steam distilled from the resin of the copaiba balsam tree
Geographic location of the plant:	Asia
Essential oil properties:	Anti-inflammatory, antibacterial
Uses:	Calms inflammation and arthritis
Body care preparation suggestions:	Lotions and salves for arthritis relief

CYPRESS ESSENTIAL OIL (*Cupressus*)
This oil gives a herbaceous, woodsy, and evergreen aroma.

Extraction process:	Steam distilled from the wood and branches of the cypress evergreen tree
Geographic location of the plant:	Mediterranean
Essential oil properties:	Fragrant, woodsy, astringent, antibacterial
Uses:	Relaxes muscles; helps with varicose veins / ruptured capillaries; relieves hemorrhoids; stimulates hair growth
Body care preparation suggestions:	Lotions and salves for sore muscles; lotions to repair varicose veins and ruptured capillaries; hair oil to stimulate growth

EUCALYPTUS ESSENTIAL OIL (*Eucalyptus globulus*)
This oil gives a camphoraceous, woodsy, and sweet aroma.

Extraction process:	Steam distilled from the leaves of the eucalyptus tree
Geographic location of the plant:	Australia
Essential oil properties:	Antiviral, antimicrobial, antibacterial
Uses:	Expands the lungs; clears nasal and chest congestion; reduces fever; repels insects
Body care preparation suggestions:	Soaps, lotions, massage oils

FENUGREEK ESSENTIAL OIL (*Trigonella foenum-graecum*)
This oil gives a mild, bittersweet, licorice-like aroma.

Extraction process:	Extracted from the seeds of the fenugreek plant
Geographic location of the plant:	South and Central Asia
Essential oil properties:	Blood sugar regulator; support for healthy testosterone levels; lactation support; anti-inflammatory; natural appetite suppressant
Uses:	Supports weight reduction; boosts metabolism; helps with appetite suppression; helps regulate blood sugar; used in Chinese medicine to treat skin conditions
Body care preparation suggestions:	Thickening agent for bath and body preparations, shampoos, conditioners, skin salves, and lotions; lactation salve

FRANKINCENSE ESSENTIAL OIL (*Boswellia sacra*)

This oil gives a rich, woodsy, and sweet aroma.

Extraction process:	Steam distilled from the tree and resin of the frankincense balsam tree
Geographic location of the plant:	Horn of Africa
Essential oil properties:	Anti-inflammatory, antiseptic, astringent, antibacterial
Uses:	Decreases the visible signs of aging; strengthens immune system; reduces blemishes; promotes intense cellular regeneration
Body care preparation suggestions:	Perfumes, masks, serums, lotions, soaps, toothpaste

GERANIUM ESSENTIAL OIL (*Pelargonium geraniaceae*)

This oil gives a sweet, herbaceous, and slightly floral aroma.

Extraction process:	Steam distilled from the geranium flower
Geographic location of the plant:	South Africa
Essential oil properties:	Antiseptic, antibacterial, antimicrobial, anti-inflammatory, aphrodisiac, antidepressant
Uses:	Reduces the appearance of scars; used in first-aid treatment; improves libido; tones skin
Body care preparation suggestions:	Natural perfumes, toners, deodorants, lotions, facial creams

GINGER ESSENTIAL OIL (*Zingiber officinale*)

This oil gives a spicy, astringent, and warm aroma.

Extraction process:	Steam distilled from the ginger root
Geographic location of the plant:	Southeast Asia
Essential oil properties:	Powerful antioxidant, circulation stimulant, fever reducer, pain reliever, nausea reducer, powerful aphrodisiac
Uses:	Fights fatigue; reduces swelling; reduces congestion; reduces spasms; helps with arthritic conditions, muscle sprains, bruising, and soreness; increases circulation; reduces fever; relieves toothaches; increases circulation; reduces nausea
Body care preparation suggestions:	Lotions, salves, perfumes, rubs

GRAPEFRUIT ESSENTIAL OIL (*Citrus paradisi*)
This oil gives a citrusy, invigorating, and sweet aroma.

Extraction process:	Cold pressed from the rind of the grapefruit
Geographic location of the plant:	Caribbean
Essential oil properties:	Antioxidant; free radical damage reduction; lymphatic drainage promotion; healthy immune system booster; astringent; disinfectant
Uses:	Reduces cellulite and tightens pores; calms acne; brightens skin; used as an astringent
Body care preparation suggestions:	Facial lotions and toners; perfumes

HELICHRYSUM ESSENTIAL OIL (*Helios asteraceae*)
This oil gives an earthy, musky, and sweet aroma.

Extraction process:	Steam distilled from helichrysum flowers
Geographic location of the plant:	Greece, Mediterranean
Essential oil properties:	Earthy, musky, and sweet; cellular regeneration stimulant, circulation stimulant, astringent, antibacterial, antimicrobial, mucolytic, vulnerary, antioxidant, antispasmodic, diuretic, expectorant, hepatic, stimulating, nervine, anti-inflammatory
Uses:	Speeds the recovery of wounds and bruises; protects the skin from ultraviolet sunrays; increases circulation, helping to remedy varicose veins, bruising, and broken capillaries; helps with acne, eczema, scar tissue, mature skin, burns, and stretch marks; reverses loose and sagging skin; relieves joint and muscle pain and spasms; encourages cellular regeneration, stimulating the production of new skin cells; increases circulation
Body care preparation suggestions:	Perfumes, soaps, lotions, salves

JASMINE ESSENTIAL OIL (*Jasminum grandiflorum*)

This oil gives a sweet, floral, and alluring aroma.

Extraction process:	Solvent extracted from jasmine flowers
Geographic location of the plant:	Himalayas, Asia
Essential oil properties:	Aphrodisiac, nervine, sedative
Uses:	Improves mood and libido; reduces depression and anxiety
Body care preparation suggestions:	Perfumes, lotions

JUNIPER BERRY ESSENTIAL OIL (*Juniperus communis*)

This oil gives a woodsy, sweet, and astringent aroma.

Extraction process:	Steam distilled from juniper berries
Geographic location of the plant:	Europe, North America, Southwest Asia
Essential oil properties:	Antiseptic, anti-inflammatory, circulatory stimulant, antiseptic, antispasmodic, diuretic, anti-toxic, nervine, antiviral, anti-infectious, anti-arthritic, detoxifier, tonic, antirheumatic
Uses:	Treats eczema, acne, cellulite, and varicose veins; used in wound care; helps reduce muscle pains and aches
Body care preparation suggestions:	Salves, rubs, astringents, toners, cellulite cream

LAVENDER ESSENTIAL OIL (*Lavandula angustifolia*)

This oil gives a floral, tranquilizing, and astringent aroma.

Extraction process:	Steam distilled from lavender flowers
Geographic location of the plant:	North Africa, Mediterranean
Essential oil properties:	Cooling, calming, relaxing, antimicrobial, sedative, antidepressant, anti-inflammatory, carminative
Uses:	Eases feelings of depression and anxiety; soothes tension; can be used in wound care
Body care preparation suggestions:	Lotions, perfumes, creams, toners, deodorants

LEMON ESSENTIAL OIL (*Rutaceae citratus*)

This oil gives a light, sweet, and citrusy aroma.

Extraction process:	Cold pressed from a lemon fruit peel
Geographic location of the plant:	Asia
Essential oil properties:	Antidepressant, anti-anxiety, purifying, astringent
Uses:	Treats oily skin; clears away impurities; tightens sagging skin and reduces cellulite; soothes muscle aches; enhances immune system functioning; enhances mood
Body care preparation suggestions:	Lotions, scrubs, perfumes

LEMONGRASS ESSENTIAL OIL (*Cymbopogon citratus*)

This oil gives an earthy, herbaceous, and citrusy aroma.

Extraction process:	Steam distilled from lemongrass in its grass form
Geographic location of the plant:	Southeast Asia
Essential oil properties:	Antifungal, antimicrobial, analgesic, antidepressant, antibacterial
Uses:	Repels insects; relieves muscle soreness; helps with jet lag
Body care preparation suggestions:	Soaps, deodorants, perfumes

LILAC ESSENTIAL OIL (*Syringa vulgaris*)

This oil gives a floral, sweet, and astringent aroma.

Extraction process:	Steam distilled from lilac blossoms
Geographic location of the plant:	Balkan Peninsula, Eastern Europe
Essential oil properties:	Astringent, anti-inflammatory, antibacterial, antifungal, heart opening, calming
Uses:	Reduces wrinkles and fine lines; eases redness and puffiness
Body care preparation suggestions:	Soaps, facial creams, perfumes, first aid

LIME ESSENTIAL OIL (*Aurantiifolia citrus*)

This oil gives an uplifting and citrusy aroma.

Extraction process:	Cold pressed from the rind of a lime fruit
Geographic location of the plant:	Southeast Asia, Northern Africa
Essential oil properties:	Cleansing, anti-anemic, antibacterial, antimicrobial, antirheumatic, anti-sclerotic, antiscorbutic, antiseptic, antispasmodic, antitoxic, antiviral, astringent, bactericidal, carminative, depurative, diaphoretic, diuretic, febrifuge, hemostatic
Uses:	Balances oily skin; fights acne; detoxifies; tightens pores; fights bacteria; calms muscle spasms; cleanses wounds; purifies air
Body care preparation suggestions:	Perfumes, lotions, toners

MARJORAM ESSENTIAL OIL (*Origanum majorana*)

This oil gives a sweet, minty, and herbaceous aroma.

Extraction process:	Steam distilled from the marjoram herb
Geographic location of the plant:	China, Egypt, Mediterranean
Essential oil properties:	Powerful antioxidant, anti-aging and anticancer agent, expectorant, antiseptic, antifungal, pain reliever, analgesic, antispasmodic, digestive, hypotensive, nervine, sedative, tonic, restorative, antibacterial
Uses:	Treats bronchitis and coughs, fungal and bacterial infections, arthritis, muscular spasms, bruises, headaches, migraines, and sore muscles; stimulates the release of serotonin; improves mood and sleep
Body care preparation suggestions:	Rubs, salves, lotions, perfumes

MELISSA ESSENTIAL OIL (*Melissa officinalis*)

This oil gives a floral, citrusy, and herbaceous aroma.

Extraction process:	Steam distilled from the flowers and leaves of the Melissa plant
Geographic location of the plant:	Europe, Asia
Essential oil properties:	Antidepressant, antispasmodic, bactericidal, carminative, cordial, diaphoretic, emmenagogue, febrifuge, hypotensive, nervine, sedative, stomachic, sudorific, tonic
Uses:	Beneficial for skin; supports a healthy immune system; has sedating effect that studies show calms the heart beat and palpitations; corrects menstrual problems; combats cold sores and fungal infections
Body care preparation suggestions:	Salves, perfume oils, lotions

MYRRH ESSENTIAL OIL (*Commiphora myrrha*)

This oil gives a musty, smoky, and dry aroma.

Extraction process:	Steam distilled from the tree and resin of the myrrh tree
Geographic location of the plant:	China, India, Middle East, Africa
Essential oil properties:	Analgesic, nervine; circulation promoter
Uses:	Improves skin by tightening pores, creating a glow, and increasing collagen production; reduces pain associated with arthritic joints; acts as a sedative, calming, and centering agent; treats indigestion, ulcers, colds, cough, asthma, lung congestion, arthritis pain, and cancer
Body care preparation suggestions:	Lotions, facial creams, perfume, tinctures, salves

OREGANO ESSENTIAL OIL (*Origanum vulgare*)
This oil gives a spicy, pungent, and herbaceous aroma.

Extraction process:	Steam distilled from the leaves and shoots of the oregano plant
Geographic location of the plant:	Europe
Essential oil properties:	Antioxidant and anti-inflammatory, analgesic, anaphrodisiac, anthelmintic, antibacterial, antifungal, anti-inflammatory, antirheumatic, antiseptic, antispasmodic, antitoxic, antiviral, aperitif, balsamic, carminative, cholagogue, choleretic, cytophylactic, diaphoretic, disinfectant, diuretic, emmenagogue, expectorant, febrifuge, hepatic, hypnotic, parasiticide, rubefacient, nerve stimulant, stomachic, sudorific, tonic, vulnerary
Uses:	Has antiviral properties that keep infections and colds at bay; reduces pain and discomfort associated with bruises, rheumatism, arthritis, ankylosis, insect bites, and even toothache pain; has antimicrobial properties that aid in the prevention of infections and elimination of fungi such as athlete's foot and lice infestation
Body care preparation suggestions:	Soaps, perfumery, incense, candles, aromatherapy

PALO SANTO ESSENTIAL OIL (*Bursera graveolens*)
This oil gives a sweet, woodsy, and warm aroma.

Extraction process:	Steam distilled from the aged wood of fallen trees
Geographic location of the plant:	Ecuador
Essential oil properties:	Anti-inflammatory, analgesic, spiritual cleansing
Uses:	Helps with concentration, focus, meditation, and artistic pursuits; reduces stress; repels insects naturally; relieves joint pain; helps with arthritis; reduces headaches and seasonal allergies; helps with nervousness and grounding
Body care preparation suggestions:	Soaps, anointing oils, lotions, body sprays

PARSLEY SEED ESSENTIAL OIL (*Petroselinum sativum*)

This oil gives a herbaceous, spicy, and warm aroma.

Extraction process:	Steam distilled from parsley herb seeds
Geographic location of the plant:	Mediterranean
Essential oil properties:	Antimicrobial, antiseptic, astringent, carminative, depurative, diuretic, emmenagogue, febrifuge, hypotensive, laxative, stimulant, stomachic, tonic, antimicrobial, detoxifying, exfoliating, antirheumatic
Uses:	Beneficial for varicose veins; increases circulation; acts as a scalp and hair tonic; calms muscle spasms; helps combat nausea
Body care preparation suggestions:	Salves, soaps, creams

PATCHOULI ESSENTIAL OIL (*Pogostemon cablin*)

This oil gives an earthy, musky, and sweet aroma.

Extraction process:	Steam distilled from the patchouli shrub
Geographic location of the plant:	China, Indonesia, India, Brazil, Malaysia
Essential oil properties:	Anti-anxiety, antidepressant, stress reliever, digestive
Uses:	Treats skin and hair ailments; stimulates cellular regeneration; reduces inflammation; promotes healthy-looking skin; treats psoriasis, eczema, acne, dandruff, and oily scalp; heals wounds; reduces appearance of scars
Body care preparation suggestions:	Cosmetic applications, personal care formulations, soaps, perfumes, incense, candles, aromatherapy

PEPPERMINT ESSENTIAL OIL (*Mentha balsamea*)

This oil gives a minty, stimulating, and cooling aroma.

Extraction process:	Steam distilled from a peppermint herb
Geographic location of the plant:	Europe, Middle East
Essential oil properties:	Analgesic, anti-inflammatory, disinfectant, antibacterial, antimicrobial, astringent, antiviral, antispasmodic, appetite suppressant
Uses:	Relieves headaches and migraines, sore muscles, and arthritic joints; reduces fever; works to suppress appetite; treats alopecia; relieves dandruff
Body care preparation suggestions:	Dental applications, shampoos, soaps, aromatherapy, insect repellent

PINE NEEDLE ESSENTIAL OIL (*Pinus sylvestris*)
This oil gives a woodsy, resinous, and pine aroma.

Extraction process:	Steam distilled from pine needles
Geographic location of the plant:	Australia
Essential oil properties:	Boosts mental, physical, and sexual energy; rejuvenative, antiphlogistic, antirheumatic, antiseptic, anti-neuralgic, antiviral, antiscorbutic, deodorant, decongestant, diuretic, disinfectant, expectorant, stimulant, tonic, antifungal
Uses:	Reduces asthma symptoms; treats bronchitis, colds, flu, sinusitis, prostatitis, arthritis, gout, sciatica, neuralgia, muscular soreness, psoriasis, eczema, ringworm, sore throat, and fever; repels insects
Body care preparation suggestions:	Oils, salves, perfume, lotions, soaps, deodorants

ROSE ESSENTIAL OIL (*Rosa damascena*)
This oil gives a deeply floral, sweet, and slightly spicy aroma.

Extraction process:	Solvent extracted from Bulgarian rose flowers
Geographic location of the plant:	Bulgaria
Essential oil properties:	Aphrodisiac, antiseptic, antispasmodic, antidepressant, anti-HIV, antioxidant, antitussive (cough suppressant), sedative; mild antiviral and antibacterial properties
Uses:	Historical: used in ancient medicine for strengthening the heart, treating menstrual bleeding, treating digestive problems, and reducing inflammation. Current: treats eczema, palpitations, and mouth infections; assists with nausea, headaches, broken capillaries, irregular menstruation, aging mature skin; balances and rejuvenates the skin; helps with impotence and nervous tension
Body care preparation suggestions:	Soaps, perfumery, incense, candles, lotions

ROSEMARY ESSENTIAL OIL (*Rosmarinus officinalis*)

This oil gives an energizing, herbaceous, and slightly citrus aroma.

Extraction process: Steam distilled from the rosemary herb

Geographic location of the plant: Spain, France, Greece, Italy

Essential oil properties: Analgesic, antirheumatic, antiseptic, astringent, antispasmodic, carminative, cytophylactic, diaphoretic, digestive, decongestant, diuretic, vulnerary, antiviral, antibacterial, antifungal, anticancer, emmenagogue, hypertensive, nervine, parasitic, restorative, tonic, circulatory stimulant

Uses: Stimulates mental cognitive processes and helps retain memory and focus; protects skin cells against the effects of ultraviolet radiation; increases blood flow; reduces blood pressure; restores strength to fragile capillaries; stimulates the growth of hair follicles and helps combat dandruff, oily hair, and premature graying; acts as a vulnerary, helping to speed recovery from wounds; assists with skin ailments such as acne, eczema, and blemishes; tones skin; tightens pores; helps with hypotension, physical fatigue, asthma, bronchitis, painful menstruation, arthritis, gout, headache, muscular soreness, bruising, cramps, weakness of limbs, varicose veins, tonsillitis, sinusitis, colds, flu, and swelling; repels insects

Body care preparation suggestions: Shampoos, conditioners, lotions, salves, perfumes

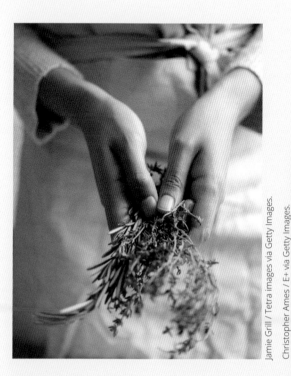

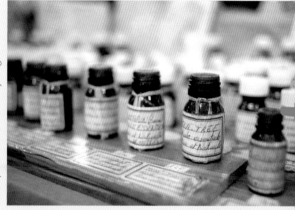

At left: Rosemary.

Essential oils in amber bottles.

Jamie Grill / Tetra images via Getty Images.

Christopher Ames / E+ via Getty Images.

ROSEWOOD ESSENTIAL OIL (*Aniba rosaeodora*)

This oil gives a floral, woodsy, and sweet aroma.

Extraction process:	Steam distilled from the wood of the rosewood tree
Geographic location of the plant:	Brazil
Essential oil properties:	Tissue regeneration
Uses:	Treats wrinkles to blemishes; can be applied without dilution; excellent for healing wounds; found in ointments
Body care preparation suggestions:	Cosmetics, personal care formulations, soaps, perfumery, incense, candles

SANDALWOOD ESSENTIAL OIL (*Santalum album*)

This oil gives a woodsy, sweet, and slightly floral aroma.

Extraction process:	Steam distilled from the wood of the sandalwood tree
Geographic location of the plant:	Australia, India
Essential oil properties:	Antiphlogistic, antiseptic, antispasmodic, aphrodisiac, astringent, diuretic, emollient, expectorant, sedative, tonic, decongestant, insecticide, anticancer, antifungal, antioxidant
Uses:	Historical: a highly revered essential oil used in India for its healing properties for more than 4,000 years; used in Chinese and Tibetan medicine as well as in ancient Egypt; used in many rituals. Current: inhibits breast cancer cells; destroys prostate cancer cells, making it useful during treatment; assists with asthma, bronchitis, acne, laryngitis, muscle spasms, varicose veins, hemorrhoids, neuralgia, respiratory infections, herpes, dry skin, and dry cough; enhances immunity; cleans the sexual organs
Body care preparation suggestions:	Face creams, lotion, salves, perfume, soaps, shampoos

SPEARMINT ESSENTIAL OIL (*Mentha spicata*)
This oil gives a strong, minty, and slightly fruity aroma.

Extraction process:	Steam distilled from the flowering spearmint plant
Geographic location of the plant:	Mediterranean
Essential oil properties:	Analgesic, anesthetic, antibacterial, anti-inflammatory, antiseptic, antispasmodic, astringent, carminative, cephalic, cholagogue, decongestant, digestive, diuretic, expectorant, febrifuge, hepatic, nervine, stimulant, stomachic, tonic
Uses:	Reduces pain and inflammation; fights infections; cleanses; soothes sore muscles; tightens pores and skin; alleviates headaches and fever; powerful antibiotic effective against staphylococcus and E. coli; treats digestive issues; eases headaches; calms nerves
Body care preparation suggestions:	Soaps, perfumes, incense, candles

SPIKENARD ESSENTIAL OIL (*Nardostachys jatamansi*)
This oil gives a rich, earthy, and penetrating aroma.

Extraction process:	Steam distilled from the root of the Spikenard plant
Geographic location of the plant:	South Asia
Essential oil properties:	Deeply relaxing and grounding, nervous system sedative, antibiotic, antifungal, anti-infectious, anti-inflammatory, antiseptic, bactericidal, deodorant, fungicidal, laxative, sedative, tonic, antioxidant
Uses:	Detoxifies the liver, fights infections, reduces inflammation
Body care preparation suggestions:	Salves, lotions, body oils

SWEET ORANGE ESSENTIAL OIL (*Citrus sinensis*)

This oil has a citrusy and sweet aroma.

Extraction process:	Cold pressed from the rind of an orange
Geographic location of the plant:	Asia
Essential oil properties:	Antibacterial; agent for clearing the lymphatic system, improving immune function
Uses:	Repels termites without the use of harmful chemicals
Body care preparation suggestions:	Soaps, perfumes, deodorants

TANGERINE ESSENTIAL OIL (*Citrus reticulata*)

This oil gives a citrusy and sweet aroma.

Extraction process:	Cold pressed from the tangerine fruit peel
Geographic location of the plant:	North Africa, Mediterranean, North America, South America
Essential oil properties:	Antiseptic, cytophylactic, anti-inflammatory, antioxidant, antispasmodic, carminative, digestive, diuretic, sedative, stimulant, tonic, antiseptic, antibacterial, antidepressant, calming
Uses:	Treats dandruff, scalp infections, acne, and stretch marks; aids in digestion; encourages creativity; induces calm; boosts metabolism; detoxifies; heals scars; purifies blood; regulates and reduces oil production in skin; boosts immunity
Body care preparation suggestions:	Lotions, salves, perfumes, scrubs, shampoos

TEA TREE ESSENTIAL OIL (*Melaleuca alternifolia*)

This oil gives a camphoraceous and astringent aroma.

Extraction process:	Steam distilled from the tree and leaves of the Melaleuca plant
Geographic location of the plant:	Australia
Essential oil properties:	Disinfectant and antifungal, powerful anti-inflammatory, disinfectant, antiviral
Uses:	Used by aboriginal peoples in Australia for thousands of years to treat insect bites, blemishes, burns, skin ailments, infected wounds, bruises, lice, dandruff
Body care preparation suggestions:	Cosmetics, soaps, perfumes, salves, incense

THYME ESSENTIAL OIL (*Thymus vulgaris ct. thymol*)
This oil gives a herbaceous, spicy, and strong aroma.

Extraction process:	Steam distilled from the leaves of the thyme plant
Geographic location of the plant:	Southern Mediterranean, North America
Essential oil properties:	Antibiotic, disinfectant, analgesic, anthelmintic, antibacterial, antifungal, anti-inflammatory, antimicrobial, antioxidant, antiseptic, antispasmodic, antiviral, bactericidal, carminative, cell proliferant, deodorant, diuretic, emmenagogue, expectorant, insecticide, parasiticide, rubefacient, stimulant, tonic, vermifuge
Uses:	Historical: used by the Egyptians in preparations for embalming the dead; burned in hospitals to stop the spread of disease; used on surgical dressings and in times of war as recently as World War I to treat battle wounds. Current: enhances the immune system and fights infection; reduces pain from sore muscles and joints; fights inflammation; cleanses and purifies; fights viruses; helps with insect bites, coughs, headaches, oily skin, itching, and poor circulation; fights odors; assists in the recovery of wounds
Body care preparation suggestions:	Lotions, salves, shampoos

TURMERIC ESSENTIAL OIL (*Curcuma longa*)
This oil gives an earthy, warm, and uplifting aroma.

Extraction process:	Steam distilled from the turmeric root
Geographic location of the plant:	India, Sri Lanka, Indonesia, China, Taiwan, Peru, Haiti, Jamaica
Essential oil properties:	Anti-inflammatory, antimicrobial, antifungal, antiseptic, analgesic, gas relieving, anti-parasitic, antiviral, antiworm
Uses:	Promotes good digestion; supports healthy liver function; prevents hair loss; reduces signs of aging in skin
Body care preparation suggestions:	Salves, ointments, lotions

VETIVER ESSENTIAL OIL (*Vetiveria zizanioides*)

This oil gives an earthy and grounding aroma.

Extraction process:	Steam distilled from the root of the vetiver plant
Geographic location of the plant:	Haiti, India, Sri Lanka, Madagascar
Essential oil properties:	Analgesic, antibacterial, antifungal, anti-inflammatory, antimicrobial, antioxidant, antiseptic, antispasmodic, depurative, emmenagogue, rubefacient, sedative, stimulant, tonic, vermifuge, vulnerary
Uses:	Heals bruises, cuts, insect bites, and stings; reverses insomnia and induces calm; relieves itching; helps with menstrual problems; soothes muscular aches and pains; reduces appearance of scars; alleviates muscle sprains and stiffness; heals wounds; eases stress by promoting tranquility and reducing anxiety
Body care preparation suggestions:	Soaps, perfume

WHITE SAGE ESSENTIAL OIL (*Salvia apiana*)

This oil gives a woodsy, herbaceous, and musky aroma.

Extraction process:	Steam distilled from the leaves of the white sage plant
Geographic location of the plant:	Mexico, United States
Essential oil properties:	Purifying, disinfectant, cleansing, calming, astringent, antiviral, antispasmodic, antimicrobial
Uses:	Ceremonial purification; aids in calming respiratory illness symptoms
Body care preparation suggestions:	Soap, shampoo, face wash, astringent

WINTERGREEN ESSENTIAL OIL (*Gaultheria fragrantissima*)
This oil gives a minty and stimulating aroma.

Extraction process:	Steam distilled from the leaves of the wintergreen plant
Geographic location of the plant:	Himalayas
Essential oil properties:	Pain reliever, antiseptic, antibacterial, antifungal, anti-inflammatory, antimicrobial, antioxidant, antiseptic, antispasmodic
Uses:	Historical: used to treat headaches, nerve pain/sciatica, arthritis, ovarian pain, and menstrual cramps. Current: relieves pain; heals skin disorders
Body care preparation suggestions:	Soaps, perfumes

YLANG YLANG ESSENTIAL OIL (*Cananga odorata*)
This oil gives a floral and sweet aroma.

Extraction process:	Steam distilled from the flowers of the ylang ylang plant
Geographic location of the plant:	South Pacific Islands
Essential oil properties:	Antiseptic, aphrodisiac, antidepressant, hypotensive, sedative, antimicrobial, euphoric, tonic, nervine, calming
Uses:	Thickens hair and stimulates hair growth; regulates oil production; moisturizes, reduces split ends; eases hypertension, palpitations and rapid breathing; pacifies acne; reduces fever; reduces stress; induces calm
Body care preparation suggestions:	Perfumes, lotions, soaps, hair and scalp oils and treatments

There are so many different ways to use essential oils in skin and hair formulations. I'll outline some of my favorite recipes in the following pages.

ROSE FACIAL TONER

Soothe and cool skin while boosting cellular regeneration with this fragrant toner, ideal for mature and sensitive skin.

WHAT YOU'LL NEED:

- 2 ounces dried organic rose petals (Note: You'll really want to go organic here, as you don't want chemical fertilizers being soaked into your skin!)
- 4 ounces witch hazel
- 20 drops rose pure essential oil

WHAT TO DO:

1. Submerge the petals in witch hazel and soak overnight in a mason jar.
2. Approximately 8 hours later, strain the petals out of the liquid, using a sieve.
3. Pour into a storage container. A glass spray bottle is best.
4. Add the rose essential oil directly to the container.

Yield:
4 ounces

Preparation time:
8 hours

Indications:
This toner moisturizes, detoxifies, promotes glowing skin, and reduces pores.

Usage:
Spritz onto your face, neck, and chest in the morning and evening following your cleansing routine.

Storage:
Store in a cool, dry place for up to 6 months.

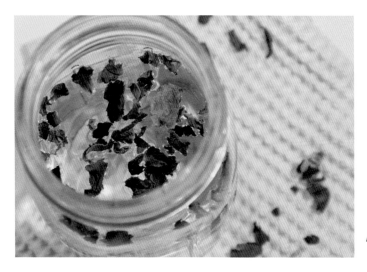

Rose Facial Toner.

TEA TREE AND PEPPERMINT MOUTHWASH

Refreshing and minty, this mouthwash will do away with the bacteria causing bad breath and tooth decay.

WHAT YOU'LL NEED:

- 1 cup distilled water
- 1 teaspoon baking soda
- 20 drops tea tree essential oil
- 10 drops peppermint essential oil

WHAT TO DO:

1. Combine the ingredients directly into a storage jar or bottle.
2. Shake vigorously until the contents are combined (the water should go from cloudy to clear).

Yield:
8 ounces

Preparation time:
5 minutes

Indications:
This mouthwash with antibacterial and antimicrobial properties freshens breath, detoxifies, and disinfects gums.

Usage:
Gargle and swish a tablespoon before brushing teeth.

Storage:
Store this mouthwash on your bathroom counter for daily use for up to 6 months.

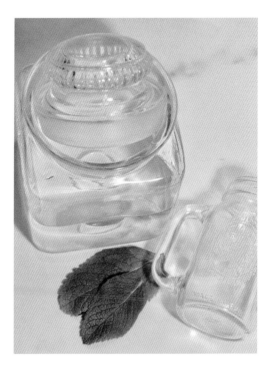

Tea Tree and Peppermint Mouthwash.

HAND SANITIZER

Moisturizing and effective, this hand sanitizer will keep you healthy between washings during cold and flu season.

WHAT YOU'LL NEED:

- ⌀ ⅛ cup rubbing (isopropyl) alcohol
- ⌀ 1 tablespoon aloe vera gel
- ⌀ 20 drops tea tree essential oil
- ⌀ 10 drops peppermint essential oil
- ⌀ 5 drops rosemary essential oil
- ⌀ 2 drops lavender essential oil

WHAT TO DO:

1. In a glass spray bottle, combine rubbing alcohol and aloe vera gel.
2. Shake this mixture vigorously to fully combine the aloe and alcohol.
3. Add the tea tree, peppermint, rosemary, and lavender essential oils and shake to combine.

Yield:
2 ounces

Preparation time:
5 minutes

Indications:
With antibacterial, antifungal, and antimicrobial properties, this hand sanitizer disinfects and leaves your skin moisturized.

Usage:
Apply a small amount to hands and rub until dissolved. Use when hands come into contact with germs.

Storage:
Take with you on the go; it will last for months.

LIP BALM

Moisturize dry, chapped lips with this soothing and long-lasting lip balm.

WHAT YOU'LL NEED:

- 1 tablespoon carnauba wax
- 3 tablespoons jojoba oil
- 1 teaspoon vitamin E oil
- 5 drops helichrysum essential oil
- 5 drops rose geranium essential oil
- 5 drops patchouli essential oil

WHAT TO DO:

1. In a double boiler (if you haven't got one, simply place a smaller pot inside a larger one containing boiling water), add 1 tablespoon carnauba wax (I used a tablespoon because I wanted a small batch) and 3 tablespoons jojoba oil.
2. Stir continuously until the wax is completely dissolved into the oil.
3. Remove your pot from the heat and add the vitamin E oil.
4. Stir the mixture and set aside to cool for 5 minutes.
5. Add essential oils and stir again.
6. Pour into a glass jar or tin for storage and let set in the refrigerator for 10 minutes.

Yield:
1½ ounces

Preparation time:
30 minutes

Indications:
This lip balm softens lips and gently exfoliates skin on lips.

Usage:
Apply a small amount to lips when needed.

Storage:
Store in a cool, dry place for up to 6 months.

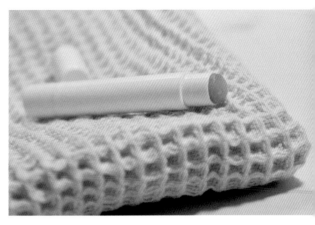

Lip Balm.

LIP GLOSS

Soften dry lips any time of the year with this easy-glide formula that can be stored in either a tin or a tube.

WHAT YOU'LL NEED:
- Beeswax
- Olive oil
- Vitamin E oil
- Essential oils of choice (I love the tingle of peppermint)
- Optional lip tint (cocoa powder, beetroot powder)

Note: Your ratio is three parts oil to one part wax.

WHAT TO DO:

1. In a double boiler (if you haven't got one, simply place a smaller pot inside a larger one containing boiling water), add 1 part beeswax (I used 1 tablespoon because I wanted a small batch) and 3 parts olive oil.
2. Stir continuously until the wax is completely dissolved into the oil. Remove the pot from the heat and add the vitamin E oil (a few drops to 1 teaspoon depending on the size of your batch).
3. Stir your mixture and set aside to cool for 5 minutes.
4. Add about 10 drops of essential oil at a 3:1 ratio measured with tablespoons (you can use this measurement to adjust for larger batches). I like the refreshing tingle of peppermint, but you can use whatever you like. Rosemary, lemon, fennel, and eucalyptus essential oils are also lovely for the lips.
5. Pour into a stick container and set in the refrigerator to solidify (10 minutes).

Yield:
This one's up to you.

Preparation time:
30 minutes

Indications:
Soothe dry, chapped lips and get a dewy sheen with this easy-to-make lip gloss.

Usage:
Apply a thin layer to lips.

Storage:
Travel sized and adaptable to various temperatures, it will last for a year.

MOISTURIZING SHAMPOO

With just enough tingle to stimulate and revitalize the scalp, this low-lather formula provides moisture as it deep cleans. This shampoo formulation is particularly great for locking moisture into curly, frizzy, and wavy hair.

WHAT YOU'LL NEED:

- ½ cup coconut milk
- ½ cup castile soap base (liquid black soap works well, too, but I prefer Dr. Bronner's Unscented baby-mild)
- 1 tablespoon coconut oil
- 1 tablespoon jojoba oil
- ½ teaspoon vitamin E oil
- 10 drops peppermint essential oil
- 20 drops tea tree essential oil

WHAT TO DO:

1. Combine the ingredients in a plastic pump bottle.
2. Give the bottle a good swirl to combine the ingredients.

Yield:
8 ounces

Preparation time:
10 minutes

Indications:
Cleansing, softening, and curl- and wave-enhancing, this shampoo leaves hair shiny and rejuvenates the scalp; the antimicrobial, antibacterial, and antifungal formula kills lice and mites.

Usage:
Apply a small amount to wet hair and lather with hands. Avoid getting in the eyes. Gentle enough for children.

Storage:
Place the bottle in the shower and enjoy the next time you wash your hair.

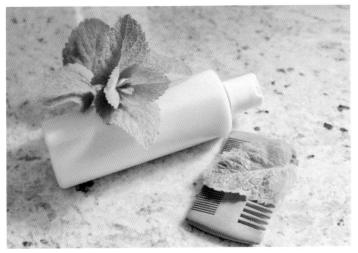

Moisturizing Shampoo with peppermint and tea tree oil.

DAILY CONDITIONER

This is a wonderful conditioner for daily use to keep tangles at bay while providing deep moisture. For fine and straight textures, apply at the ends of hair to protect against split ends. For curly hair textures, apply liberally from root to end and hand detangle or use a wide-tooth comb.

WHAT YOU'LL NEED:

- 6 tablespoons unrefined coconut oil
- 2 tablespoons olive oil
- 2 tablespoons castor oil
- 1 teaspoon vitamin E oil
- 20 drops myrrh essential oil
- 15 drops lavender essential oil
- 10 drops ylang ylang essential oil

WHAT TO DO:

1. I combine my ingredients directly in my storage container. If your coconut oil is hard, soften it by running the jar under warm water so that the items blend easily and evenly.
2. Mix with a small whisk and ta-da!

Yield:
4 ounces

Preparation time:
10 minutes

Indications:
This moisturizing, protective, softening, and aromatic conditioner promotes healthy scalp and hair growth.

Usage:
Apply a liberal amount to hair after washing or use alone on wet hair. Let sit on hair for 5 minutes before rinsing.

Storage:
Store in a cool, dry place for up to 6 months.

CLOVE MOUTHWASH

This antimicrobial mouthwash is designed to address oral discomfort, as it provides a temporary numbing sensation, making it an effective way to manage (in the short term) oral inflammation, cavity pain, and root canal pain. In addition to its analgesic properties, it will clean the mouth and leave it smelling fresh.

WHAT YOU'LL NEED:

- 1 cup purified water
- 1 heaping teaspoon ground cloves
- ¼ teaspoon sea salt
- 10 drops clove essential oil
- 5 drops tea tree essential oil

WHAT TO DO:

1. Bring 1 cup of purified water to a boil.
2. Add the cloves and sea salt and reduce to a simmer for 15 minutes.
3. Allow the pot of water to cool until lukewarm.
4. Pour into a mason jar, using a coffee filter to strain the cloves.
5. Add the clove and tea tree essential oils to the strained mixture in your mason jar and shake vigorously.

Yield:
4 ounces

Preparation time:
45 minutes

Indications:
Soothing and pacifying, this clove-based mouthwash, in addition to being used as a regular preventative, is ideal for anyone dealing with acute oral discomfort, inflammation, and root or cavity pain between dentist visits.

Usage:
Gargle twice daily as you would with regular mouthwash.

Storage:
Store in the refrigerator for up to 6 weeks. Remove from the refrigerator 30 minutes before use.

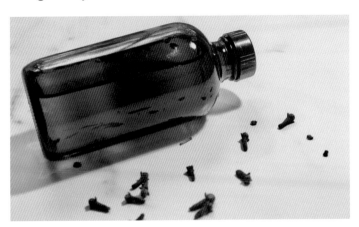

Clove Mouthwash.

ESSENTIAL OIL DEODORANT BLEND

Fragrant, gentle, and so easy to apply, this essential oil deodorant blend, designed for roller bottle application, will leave you fresh and aromatized all day long.

WHAT YOU'LL NEED:

- Fractionated coconut oil
- White thyme essential oil
- Tea tree essential oil
- Rose essential oil
- Rose geranium essential oil
- Ylang ylang essential oil
- Lavender essential oil
- Vegetable glycerin (a few drops)

WHAT TO DO:

1. Combine all ingredients in a storage jar. The amount of each ingredient is dependent upon the size of the storage jar, so you can reference the Deodorant Blending Guide (below) to help determine the proper ratio. Add a few drops of vegetable glycerin and shake.

Yield:
Dependent upon the size of the roller container

Indications:
Fragrant and uplifting, this essential oil deodorant blend is an excellent all-natural option that is particularly well suited for the wintertime when perspiration is at a minimum.

Usage:
Roll underneath arms as needed.

Storage:
Store in a cool, dry place in an amber or cobalt glass roller container for up to a year.

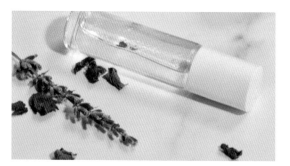

Essential Oil Deodorant Blend.

Deodorant Blending Guide

Blending essential oils isn't an exact science. Approximate how much you'll need to satisfy your percentage based on the size of your container. When you're finished, add a few drops (usually between 5 and 7 drops if you're working with a standard ½-ounce roller container) of vegetable glycerin and shake.

Fractionated coconut oil	10%	Mixture of ½ rose and ½ rose geranium essential oil	20%
White thyme essential oil	10%	Ylang ylang essential oil	20%
Tea tree essential oil	10%	Lavender essential oil	30%

MOISTURIZING BODY WASH

Gentle enough for sensitive and children's skin, this fragrant and moisturizing body wash will remove dirt and grime to reveal soft, supple skin.

WHAT YOU'LL NEED:

- ½ cup castile soap
- 4 tablespoons vegetable glycerin
- ½ teaspoon vitamin E oil
- 4 tablespoons olive oil
- 15 drops bergamot essential oil
- 10 drops rosemary essential oil
- 5 drops peppermint essential oil

WHAT TO DO:

1. In a measuring cup, measure out the castile soap. Add the vegetable glycerin and whisk or stir.
2. Then add the vitamin E and olive oils, and whisk or stir once again.
3. Finally, add any essential oils.

Yield:
8 ounces

Indications:
Safe for sensitive skin, this nondrying and calming body wash gently cleanses, revitalizes skin, and stimulates circulation.

Usage:
Apply a small amount to wet skin. This formulation lathers very well. A little bit goes a long way.

Storage:
Store in a cool, dry place.

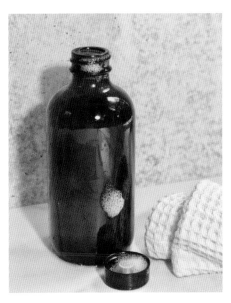

Moisturizing Body Wash.

ALOE VERA
COSTA RICA

Central America, Summer 2009

I was assigned the obstinate horse. Instead of taking the charted course, walking single file along the volcanic trail like every other self-respecting horse in the group, my horse was a galloper, a sprinter, who preferred to take the path untrodden. I was visiting my friend Liza, who was teaching English in San José, Costa Rica. After spending a week in the capital city, we were off to explore.

Our first stop was Arenal, the northern town that boasted waterfalls and the stunning Arenal Volcano, before eventually making our way across the border to Nicaragua for a few days. We took a rickety bus crowded with backpackers and locals from San José to Arenal. The drive was scenic as the landscape—overcast, green, and increasingly mountainous—extended before us. The earth, soft, looked like ground charcoal as we made our way by foot from the bus stop to the sleepy town. Without much effort, we found a beautiful little hostel high in the mountains to set up camp for the next few days.

We planned to take a tour of the Arenal Volcano, one of the town's biggest draws, but shortly after our lunch at a roadside stand, Liza, who had ordered chicken and rice instead of the vegetarian plantain and queso mash that I had enjoyed, came down with a case of food poisoning. By that evening, it was clear that she wasn't in any shape to go sightseeing, so I headed out solo the next morning for my horseback tour of the Arenal Volcano. I rose with the sun and made my way to the courtyard behind the hostel's front gate to be picked up and eventually shuttled off into the luminous sunrise toward the horse ranch.

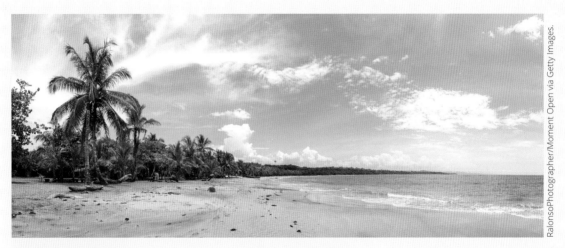

Caribbean coast.

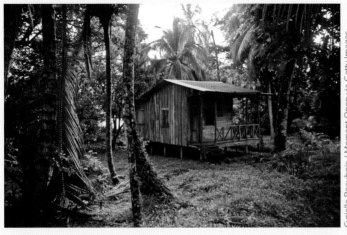

Cabin in the forest, Costa Rica.

At right: Arenal Volcano, Costa Rica.

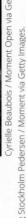

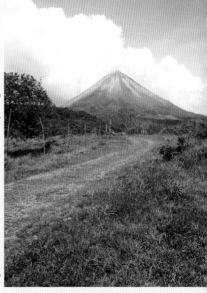

The air was thin and dry in the mountains. Lush vegetation, almost rainforest-like, surrounded us. Ours was a medium-sized tour group of mostly European tourists from Italy. Of the many languages that circled around me, English wasn't one. I focused instead—and with much relief—on the lush landscape, since small talk wasn't in the cards. We saddled our horses and were off. The riding trail cut through a golden open plain, the coveted Arenal Volcano hazy in the distance. The plan was to ride to the volcano, let the horses carry us partially up a trail leading to the waterfall, get off the horses, and hike the rest of the way to the mouth of the waterfall, where we could swim and relax before hiking back to the horses.

My horse, the wily one, was in the lead. I was even in front of the guide, who on several occasions had to race up to me and grab hold of the reins to redirect my stubborn four-legged friend. I remember vividly the wild twitch of his ears, the way his head bobbed up and down as if he were trying to free himself of the bit inside his mouth. To say that my life didn't flash before my eyes on several occasions would be a lie; however, the silver lining was that, being in front, I had the perfect, uninterrupted view of the splendor that lay before me. I reveled in the way the morning light danced golden and peach across the open green field, the purple and blue smoky hues of the volcano in the distance, and the beautiful intricacy of the rainforest around us and the various shades of green that radiated from within. The landscape was wild and stunning, unlike anything I'd seen before. The call of the forest was primal and vibrational. My horse must have heard what I heard because he kept racing away from the narrow dirt path toward the forests, bewitched by the strange songs of howler monkeys and tree frogs. Wind in my face, I embraced each bump as we made our way toward the majestic purple volcano.

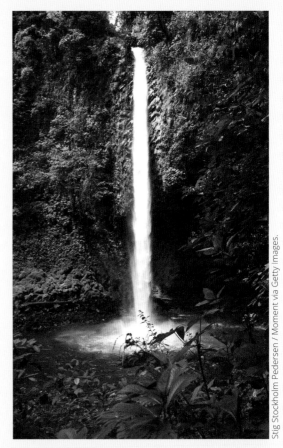

Arenal Waterfall, Costa Rica.

Stig Stockholm Pedersen / Moment via Getty Images.

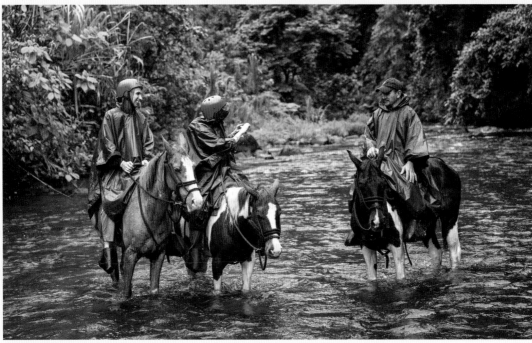

Arenal horseback trek.

DavorLovincic / E+ via Getty Images.

Once on the volcano's path, the temperature dropped, and the sunlight became overcast by a tangle of vines and palms. On several occasions, I had to duck to avoid being hit in the head by a branch. The primitive song of the earth's beating heart grew louder and louder as bugs and birds joined the chorus of frogs and monkeys. The higher we trekked, the greener and cooler it became; the air transitioned into a humid, earthy force as the trees grew taller, more elaborate, as if the volcanic soil possessed a certain magic that garnered a superior stock of tree, one with artistic vines twisting and coiling.

Every plant looked exotic, unfamiliar, and vibrant. There were so many shades and textures: waxy green leaves, dripping wet with jungle dew, and fuzzy, sage-colored plants, with resting bugs nestled to their bosoms. I recognized a seductive bird of paradise here, some lace-patterned ferns there, and then I had to blink several times to process the absolutely enormous aloe plants that seemed to grow alongside the mountain. Fat and juicy looking, they were the very picture of aloe perfection. They were nothing like the aloes I was familiar with in New York,

the finicky little succulents that drooped and sagged moodily on my window ledge despite how much I did or didn't water them or how much sun they did or didn't get. These aloes were very different. Wild and free, they were bursting, plump with serum; it dawned on me that I was seeing aloe plants in their natural environment for the first time, and it was spectacular.

Before long, I was walking through the forest on foot, making my way toward the La Fortuna Waterfall. My flip-flopped feet (not the best shoe choice, I'll admit) sank into the rich black soil, sliding occasionally as I progressed uphill. As I sat on a slick black rock at the base of the volcano, I closed my eyes; the mist from the water settled onto my skin, and the sound of the waterfall purified and calmed my soul. It was such a stroke of luck that I, the only English speaker, away from the rest of the group, was able to have a truly private moment to myself in the bosom of the earth. The water was exceptionally purifying, but so, too, were the plants. If the color green had an odor, it was present in the air that morning. In my mind, I couldn't shake the vision of the aloe plants I'd seen.

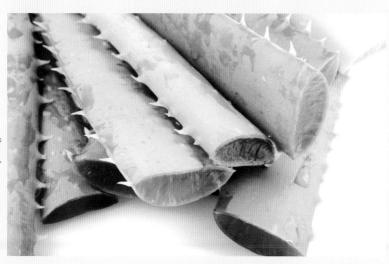

Nenov/Moment via Getty Images.

Aloe vera plant cuttings.

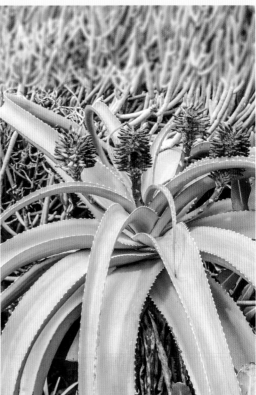

Arenal Volcano.

During our ride back to the horse ranch, I asked my guide (who by then had resigned himself to holding my horse's reins in his left hand and his horse's reins in his right hand) about the aloe plants. He didn't have much to say about the cosmetic and healing properties of aloe, but he spoke enthusiastically about aloe juice and told me about a stall at the market that sold "the purest" aloe juice. Aloe, he promised, would cleanse my body of any ailments. I thought about Liza, sick at the hostel with food poisoning, and though I never did make it to the market in Arenal or taste the reputed curative aloe juice, I shared my newfound information about the healing benefits of aloe vera. In the quiet of the afternoon, I rocked in a hammock in the courtyard of the hostel, journal in hand, brainstorming ways to incorporate aloe vera in bath and body formulations.

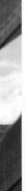

Wild aloe vera, Arenal, Costa Rica.

ALOE VERA 100%

Antioxidant rich, aloe gel is full of enzymes that help exfoliate and cool the skin. Aloe vera is a natural moisturizer that calms the skin without leaving it oily. Its other benefits include the following:

- Anti-inflammatory properties
- Cooling and calming
- Deeply moisturizing
- Rich in vitamins A and C
- May help prevent wrinkles and the appearance of scars
- Soothes burns and minor scrapes
- Relieves dandruff

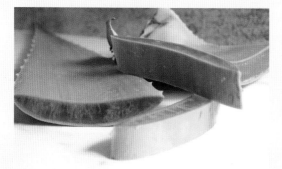

Sliced aloe.

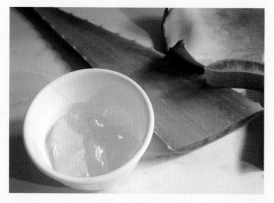

Aloe vera gel.

In ancient China, aloe vera was used to moisturize and soften skin. Cleopatra is rumored to have used aloe vera on her skin and hair. Native Americans used aloe vera to protect their skin from insect bites and then to treat the bites. There are so many different ways to use aloe vera in skin and hair formulations. I'll outline some of my favorite recipes on the following pages.

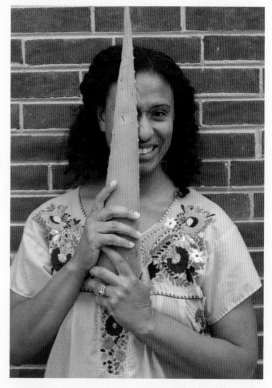

This large aloe leaf can supply gel for more than a dozen products.

SCALP-REJUVENATING SERUM

This lightweight and cooling serum will gently exfoliate while cleansing the scalp to encourage hair growth, treat dandruff, and encourage optimal circulation.

WHAT YOU'LL NEED:

- 1 tablespoon aloe vera gel
- 1 teaspoon black castor oil
- 1 teaspoon black seed oil
- 4 drops tea tree essential oil
- 2 drops peppermint essential oil

WHAT TO DO:

1. Mix the aloe vera gel, black castor oil, and black seed oil together until combined smoothly.
2. Add the tea tree oil and peppermint oil.

Yield:
One 1-ounce amber jar

Preparation time:
5 minutes

Indications:
This serum with antimicrobial and antibacterial properties soothes, moisturizes, and stimulates hair growth.

Usage:
Apply to a moist or dry scalp 2–3 times a week before styling.

Storage:
Store in a cool, dry place for up to 3 months.

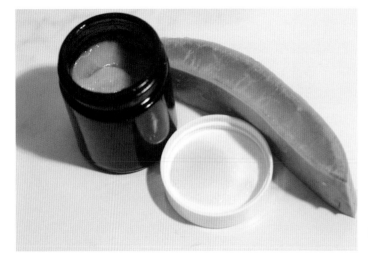

Scalp-Rejuvenating Serum.

MOISTURIZING ALOE VERA FACE MASK

Restore your skin's natural balance with this gentle, softening, and soothing gel face mask.

WHAT YOU'LL NEED:

- 2 tablespoons aloe vera gel
- 1 tablespoon raw honey
- 1 tablespoon jojoba oil

WHAT TO DO:

1. Either scrape the gel from a large aloe vera leaf or use organic aloe vera gel.
2. Mix the aloe vera gel with the honey and jojoba oil.

Yield:
One 2-ounce container

Preparation time:
10 minutes

Indications:
This calming, cooling, and soothing face mask also reduces inflammation.

Usage:
Apply to a clean, dry face. Leave on for 10 minutes, and then rinse.

Storage:
Store in a cool, dry place.

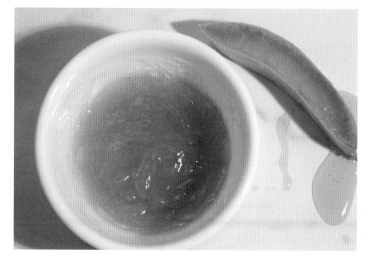

Moisturizing Aloe Vera Face Mask.

HAIR CONDITIONING MASK

This is a wonderful before-shower hair-strengthening treatment for all hair types. Aloe moisturizes and strengthens the hair shaft, protecting your locks from heat, environmental, and style damage.

WHAT YOU'LL NEED:

- 2 ounces aloe vera gel

WHAT TO DO:

1. Scrape about 2 ounces of aloe vera gel from a large aloe vera leaf or use organic aloe vera gel.

Yield:
2 ounces

Preparation time:
5 minutes

Indications:
This gel conditions and moisturizes hair and seals the hair shaft.

Usage:
Apply gel to clean, wet hair from root to tip. Wrap your hair in a towel and wait for 20 minutes. Rinse and condition as usual.

Storage:
Store excess gel in an airtight container in a cool, dry place for up to 6 weeks.

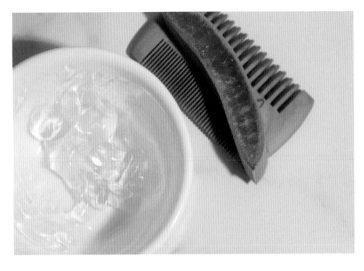

Hair Conditioning Mask.

DETANGLING HAIR SERUM

This detangling serum works wonders on freshly washed and/or conditioned hair. Light and nongreasy, this gel will moisturize locks while leaving hair manageable and easy to brush or comb.

WHAT YOU'LL NEED:

- 1 tablespoon aloe vera gel
- ⅛ teaspoon vegetable glycerin
- 2 drops lavender essential oil
- ½ teaspoon black castor oil

WHAT TO DO:

1. Mix ingredients together.

Yield:
1½ ounces

Preparation time:
10 minutes

Indications:
This serum detangles, softens, conditions, and moisturizes hair.

Usage:
Section your hair into quadrants, or any other manageable portions. Apply the detangling serum to wet hair, starting at the root and moving down the hair shaft to the ends.

Storage:
Store in an amber or cobalt jar in a cool, dry place for up to 6 months. Try not to get moisture from your hands into the jar, as it will reduce the shelf life if water is introduced.

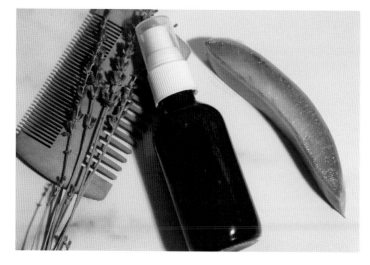

Detangling Hair Serum.

WHIPPED ALOE VERA LOTION

This is an ultra-light whipped body lotion, ideal for summertime or after-sun applications.

WHAT YOU'LL NEED:

- ¼ cup aloe vera gel
- ¼ cup coconut oil (softened)
- ¼ cup shea butter
- 1 teaspoon vegetable glycerin
- ⅛ teaspoon vitamin E oil
- 5 drops essential oil of choice

WHAT TO DO:

1. With a hand mixer, blend the aloe vera gel until it's white.
2. Melt the shea butter in a double boiler over low heat or by using a Pyrex glass container placed inside a pot filled with about 2 inches of boiling water.
3. If your coconut oil is hard, soften it by running the jar under warm water. Fold in softened coconut oil, shea butter, vegetable glycerin, and vitamin E oil.
4. Whip until light and creamy.
5. Add 5 drops of essential oil of choice.
6. Hand blend again to a whipped consistency.

Yield:
6 ounces

Preparation time:
30 minutes

Indications:
This light, moisturizing, and nongreasy lotion absorbs easily into skin.

Usage:
Apply as often as needed. Suitable for face and body.

Storage:
Store in a cool, dry place for up to 6 months.

LAVENDER ALOE SALVE

This cooling salve can serve as a spot treatment for inflammatory skin conditions like acne or minor burns. For facial applications, this salve works well after washing or toning. The salve can also be applied directly to minor abrasions and scrapes.

WHAT YOU'LL NEED:

- Medium aloe trimming
- 5 drops lavender essential oil

WHAT TO DO:

1. First, cut off a section of the aloe trimming. I took from the widest point to yield the most gel. Cut the leaf in half and allow the aloe gel and juice to drip into a jar.
2. Once full of aloe vera gel, add 5 drops of lavender essential oil. Cap the jar and give it a good shake to mix.

Yield:
One ½-ounce container

Preparation time:
10 minutes

Indications:
This antibacterial, calming, and cooling salve also reduces inflammation.

Uses:
Apply to bruises, sore muscles, scrapes, acne, and minor skin irritations.

Storage:
Store in a cool, dry place for up to 6 months.

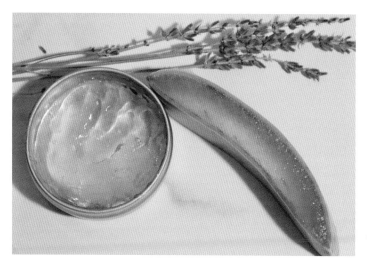

Lavender Aloe Salve.

VINEGAR EXTRACTIONS
JAPAN

East Asia, Spring 2012

We were moving so quickly, so smoothly, that it felt as though we were suspended in midair, perfectly still. It's what I imagine it must be like in the eye of a tornado. Only my husband, son, and I were riding the bullet train, an experience that was like a meditation in and of itself. It was easy to forget how fast we were going—a reported 200 miles per hour. Mark, my jazz musician husband, was on tour, and our two weeks in Tokyo had come to a close. We were now on our way to Osaka, but first we were to stop in Kyoto.

Tokyo blew me away at first. As a New Yorker, it was jaw dropping to step into a much larger and busier city. The buildings, astonishing modern marvels, were taller and sleeker than the skyscrapers I'd left behind. My jaw dropped at the sheer pleasantness and efficiency of everything. Despite being an enormous and crowded city, Tokyo was clean—no, not clean, pristine. I might be tempted to actually use the 10-second rule if food dropped to the ground. Tokyo was civil, polite, orderly, and quiet. People left unchained bicycles unattended while they worked with the full knowledge and expectation that they'd be there at the end of the day. There was no dashing across the street to make the light, no honking aggressive drivers, and no panhandlers, roaches, or rats. Classical music and nature sounds streamed from the Metro during peak rush hour. There was a feeling of Zen and balance everywhere.

But it was toward the end of the first week, after the shine of the neon lights in the Kabukicho light district in Shinjuku and the dazzle of technology that was not yet available in the United States in the Akihabara district began to wear off, that I began to reflect on my time in Tokyo. From the complexity of making my way across

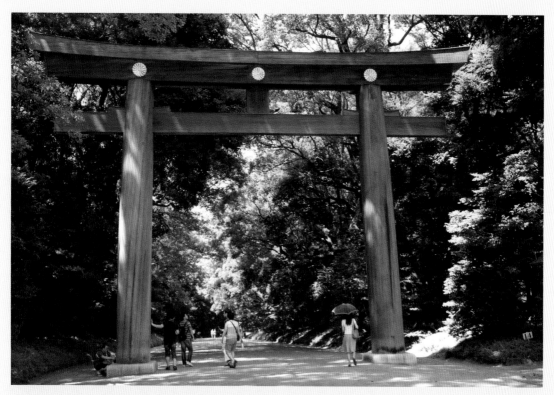

Ready for a forest bath at a Tokyo shrine.

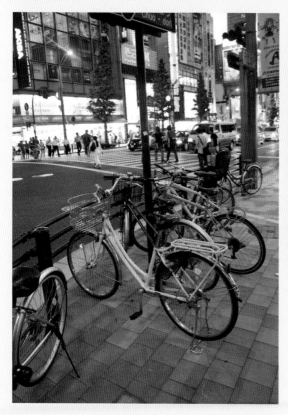

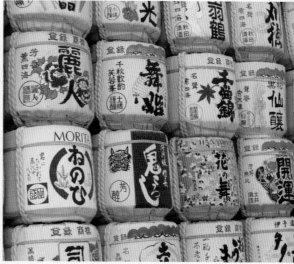

Saki barrels, Tokyo, Japan.

At left: The serene bustle of Tokyo, Japan.

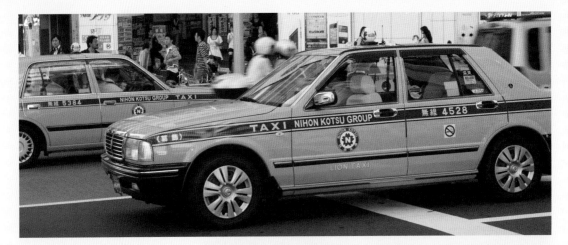

On the go in Tokyo, Japan.

At right: Bamboo garden, Tokyo, Japan.

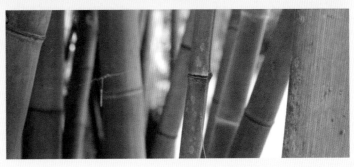

the famed Shibuya crossing right outside the doors of our hotel to wandering the beautifully manicured gardens outside of the Imperial Palace, I was aware that I was in Japan, but I didn't feel necessarily like I had left New York. Though we had our fair share of traditional sushi, sashimi, and ramen, Tokyo was so full of fine French and Italian dining, delectable French pastries, ice cream and crepe trucks, classical music, and cutting-edge modernity that it was often hard to place where I was. It was only during my forest baths and visits to the stunning Zen and Buddhist shrines and temples that I felt a true and unmistakable sense of Japan.

I had the pleasure of touring the Meiji-jingu Shrine, Yasakuni-jinja Shrine, Toshogu-jinga Shrine, and Nogi-jinja Shrine. These forested retreats, tucked away in the heart of the city, were cocoons

of calm. I wanted to experience more of this effect, which is why the idea of the ancient and forested city of Kyoto thrilled me so. That and the fact that Mark, who had been to Tokyo probably 30 times already, had never been, and it would be a part of Japan we could discover together.

The bullet train slipped into the Kyoto station, coming to the smoothest and cleanest halt. Mark gathered our things as I tightened the harness I was using to carry our very Zen little one-year-old, who seemed to be experiencing Japan with the same wide-eyed wonder that I felt. We made our way onto the platform and then followed the signs to the famous Rokuon-ji Zen Buddhist temple. It was the perfect spring day—warm enough to take off our sweaters but decidedly overcast. The air in Kyoto had a different energy. It was more humid, felt somehow ancient, and carried the fragrant, subtle aroma of cherry blossom flowers—an aroma, to be honest, that sent me into several acute sneezing attacks. In the distance were majestic rolling woodland hills. Pale pink, cherry blossoms lined the streets. And before us, the golden Rokuon-ji temple glimmered in the cloud-filtered sunlight.

We had arrived, serendipitously, at the peak of Sakura (cherry blossom) season. Women dressed as geishas walked gracefully down the pink-petaled paths, cherry blossom petals standing out like snowflakes against their dark hair. The shops lining the street sold every imaginable cherry blossom souvenir, but what held my attention even more than the beautiful framed prints that I purchased were the discreet slender bottles of cherry blossom plum vinegar. I had never heard of it, and, always on the lookout for new natural products, I had so many questions for the patient shop owners.

Cherry blossom plum vinegar was a vinegar made from cherry blossom extract, and it was often used in Japanese skin care products to smooth skin texture due to its anti-aging properties. Cherry blossom plum vinegar is rich in caffeic acid and phenolic antioxidants, making it regenerative, anti-inflammatory, anti-aging, clarifying, and collagen promoting, resulting in a smooth, clear, hydrated, and even complexion. Cherry blossom extract heals irritated skin and reduces redness.

At home in New York, I had just begun exploring the use of apple cider vinegar on my skin as a toner and loved the results, so I was excited to try cherry blossom plum vinegar. For centuries, vinegar has been used as more than a mere dressing for salad. Vinegar has been used on skin and hair to clear dandruff, exfoliate, balance pH, and soothe inflammation. The ancient Greeks used vinegar to wash their hands and faces and as a mouth gargle. In medieval times, vinegar was used as a facial astringent; additionally, oatmeal boiled in vinegar was used to clear skin. The boiled oatmeal addition dried oily skin and assisted in the natural exfoliation process of the vinegar. In 17th-century France, perfumes and smelling liquids were made out of floral-infused vinegars.

There are so many different ways to use vinegar in skin and hair formulations. I'll outline some of my favorite recipes in the following pages.

The Golden Shrine.

Below: The Golden Temple, Kyoto, Japan.

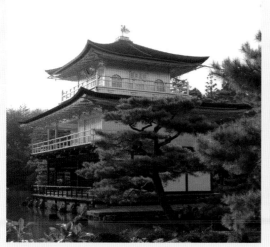

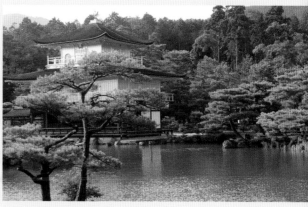

RASPBERRY VINEGAR TONER

Reduce shine, control oil, and calm acne with this clarifying toner.

WHAT YOU'LL NEED:

- ¼ cup raspberry vinegar
- ¼ cup strongly brewed organic green tea

WHAT TO DO:

1. Bring your tea water to boil; for ¼ cup of boiling water, steep two bags of organic green tea for 20 minutes.
2. Remove the tea bags or loose tea.
3. Let green tea cool.
4. Pour your tea into a spray bottle and add the raspberry vinegar.

Yield:
One 4-ounce spray jar

Preparation time:
25 minutes

Indications:
With antibacterial properties, this calming and clarifying toner also regulates oil production.

Usage:
Apply as a spray or with a cotton ball to a clean face once or twice daily.

Storage:
Store in the refrigerator for up to 6 weeks.

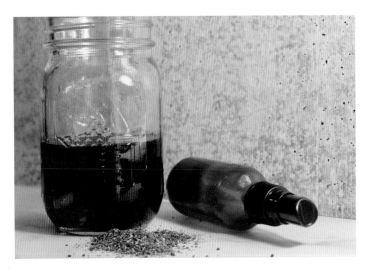

Raspberry Vinegar Toner.

CHERRY BLOSSOM VINEGAR TONER

Age gracefully with this antioxidant-packed toner. Ideal for maturing/mature skin, this toner will brighten, smooth, plump, and reduce the appearance of wrinkles.

WHAT YOU'LL NEED:

- ¼ cup cherry blossom vinegar
- ¼ cup rosewater

WHAT TO DO:

1. Combine the cherry blossom vinegar and rosewater.

Yield:
One 4-ounce spray bottle

Preparation time:
5 minutes

Indications:
With anti-aging and antioxidant properties, this soothing and calming toner brightens and clarifies skin while reducing the appearance of wrinkles and fine lines.

Usage:
Apply as a spray or on a cotton ball to a clean face once or twice daily.

Storage:
Store in a cool, dry place for up to 6 months.

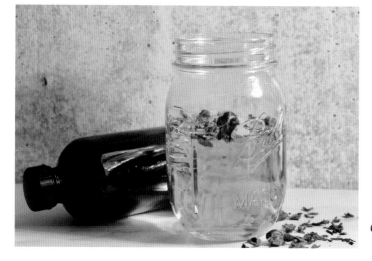

Cherry Blossom Vinegar Toner.

RICE VINEGAR TONER

Perfect for sensitive skin, this rice vinegar toner is cooling and pacifying.

WHAT YOU'LL NEED:

- ⅛ cup strongly brewed organic mint tea
- ¼ cup rice vinegar
- ⅛ cup witch hazel

WHAT TO DO:

1. Steep an organic mint tea bag in ⅛ cup of boiling water for 20 minutes.
2. Remove the tea bag and let the tea water cool.
3. Once the tea is cool, combine it with the rice vinegar and witch hazel.

Yield:
One 4-ounce jar

Preparation time:
30 minutes

Indications:
With astringent properties, this toner tightens skin and pores, clarifies, and smooths the surface appearance of skin.

Usage:
Apply as a spray or on a cotton ball to a clean face once or twice daily.

Storage:
Store in the refrigerator for up to 6 weeks.

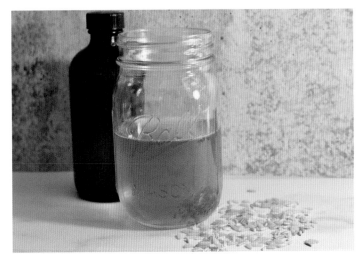

Rice Vinegar Toner.

PLANT BARKS
MOZAMBIQUE

Southeastern Africa, 2007–2008

I taught the late class. It was a time slot nobody wanted, and since I was the most recent hire at the teacher training college where I worked in Inhambane, Mozambique, it became my time slot. It was an open-format English as a Second Language (ESL) course geared toward the teachers in training so that they could lead effective English language classes for their primary school–aged students.

The truth was that most of the teachers were fluent in English already. They were much more fluent in English than I was in Portuguese, and our conversations were a curious combination of the two languages. For the purposes of my Monday evening ESL class, we began with a unit on songs. Music had such universal appeal, and my students, I quickly learned, were enormous Bob Marley fans. We would spend hours in our small pink-painted cement classroom, as the sun went down, reading and pronouncing lyrics and singing and dissecting the song lineup from the *Bob Marley Greatest Hits* album. It was so much fun. These future teachers were the most enthusiastic students I'd ever had the privilege to teach. I don't even have enough time to describe the pure joy I saw on the faces of their primary school–aged students, sometimes crammed 70 to a classroom, seated on the floor, as they sang the songs we'd practiced in class the week before. My field observations were so precious.

At 9:00 p.m., our Monday night class was dismissed. We always left together. My students were so thoughtful to help me tidy up and close down the classroom. Once we'd swept and wiped the desks, grabbed our bags, and turned out the lights, we would make our way down

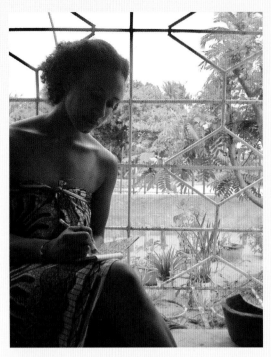

Journaling on my patio in Inhambane, Mozambique.

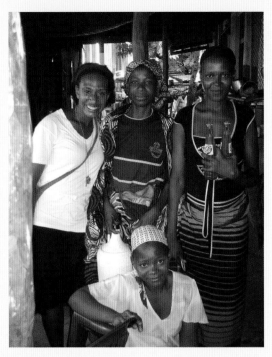

With the chefs at a restaurant in the Central Market in Inhambane, Mozambique.

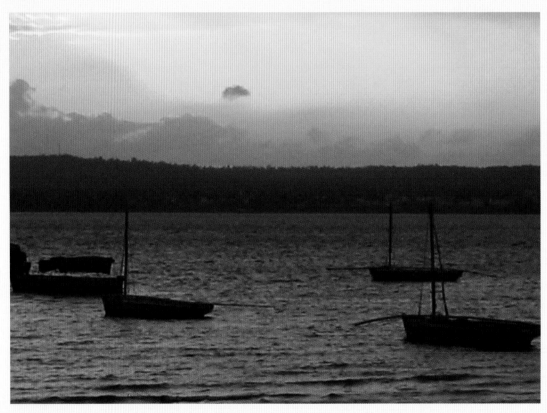

Fishing boats in Inhambane Bay, Mozambique.

the cool open air breezeway that connected the classrooms to the one and only path through the tall grass that led to the main road.

I was never so in tune with the rhythms of the moon as I was while living in Mozambique. I lived and worked in rural Inhambane, an oceanside southern province not far from the South African border. In the small sandy village where I worked, there were few street lights. In fact, there were none. No street lights. No reflective signs. The only lights you would see while making your way home came from either a light inside a house you passed along the way or the moon. When the moon was full, the sky opened up, radiating a light so brilliant you could see all of the shapes around you and well into the distance. I loved these nights, everything bathed in an indigo glow. But when the moon was not visible in the sky, it was pitch black. You were hard pressed to see your hand if you held it up directly in front of your face. It took me months to get used to this new reality; I was terrified I'd walk into a spider web (and trust me, those spiders were not small), a swarm of bats, a wild animal (this was the Southern African brush), or, worse yet, a serial killer (the least likely scenario; yet my vigilant and paranoid New York self was always prepared for the worst case, just in case). Little did I know that the worst case, which I'd soon encounter, couldn't have been further from the form of any of the above scenarios.

On this particular night, there was no moon. The sky was a dark cloak. It had been overcast during the day from the heavy morning rain. Even the stars, which were usually on bright display, seemed to be in hiding. It was, after all, cyclone season. In a single-file line, we walked one by one through the path in the grass. The voices in front of me and behind me, and the sensation of grass on my ankles and shins, were my only guides as my flip-flopped feet waited to connect with the dirt road, my cue to cross the street and turn right.

At the dirt road, we said our "Ate logos" and "Boa noites" and began to disperse. The majority of my students went to the left toward the dormitories, while I had about a half mile walk ahead of me to the right, as I lived in a small house off campus situated toward the back of the property that housed the stately home of the school director. One foot in front of the other, keeping to the very edge of the dirt road, the tall grass to my left, I made my way toward the small cluster of homes that made up the neighborhood where I lived.

The night was humid and still, and crickets sang from their hideouts between the blades of grass. From time to time, I'd hear the squeaky wheels of a bicyclist and the familiar "Ola" ("Hello") or "Boa tarde, Professora" ("Good afternoon, Teacher") called out in greeting. I could never quite figure out how everyone who passed in the pitch darkness, people whom I certainly couldn't make out, seemed to know it was me, but there was a great comfort in the anonymous knowing.

Finally, I made it to my turn off. There was a cluster of palm trees under which one of our neighbors always parked a white pickup truck. I made my way slowly from the red dirt road to the sandy path that led to my home. I passed the small shop stand where fruit, digestive biscuits, soda, and beer were sold. It was closed and boarded up for the evening, but it was a useful landmark. At last I could see the kitchen and living room light from my neighbor's house. I made it to my teal-colored cement porch. As usual, the housekeeper had not left the light on for me. "Wasteful," she would scold. It was a fight I'd given up long ago. I fished through my bag for my keys and felt for the door-knob and then the small slit that indicated a keyhole. Door open, I turned on the light and made my way into the kitchen and living room, which were adjoined. I tossed my bag onto the sofa, picked up my flash-light (which I had forgotten to bring with me to work), and made my way—after flipping on the porch lights—outside again and toward the communal outdoor bath-rooms shared by the cluster of houses where I lived. We all shared a backyard, which held a well for fetching water, a clothesline, a shower hut, and two bath-room huts.

After using the bathroom, I made my way back into the house, where I washed my hands and face and brushed my teeth in the water basin the housekeeper had set out. The water, which had been boiled late that afternoon before she left, was still warm. Ready for bed, I went into my bedroom and immediately noticed some-thing out of place.

At first I was confused. It took me a while to process what I was seeing. It was as if I was looking at a black furry rug along the bottom of the wall where it met the floor near my desk. I took a step closer, and my heart began to pound—it wasn't a rug. It wasn't a rug at all; it was a spider. It was an enormous spider, the size of a small toy lapdog, clinging to the wall in my room. I felt my eyes widen in horror; I covered my mouth to muffle my scream. My entire body began to shake. It was literally the largest spider I had ever

seen, including large scary spiders behind glass tanks at the zoo. It was larger than a tarantula.

Naively, I ran into the kitchen to grab my can of Baygonne (the Mozambican equivalent of RAID), which worked on most local spiders the size of my hand and smaller. But when I sprayed this crea-ture, my attempt to kill it only made it angry—very angry. The spiders in Mozam-bique were enormous and imposing, and this was the worst and largest I'd ever seen. Later I'd learn that I was face-to-face with a giant huntsman spider. These spiders were the worst! They came with the strangest feature. They'd lay flat and crablike, in what I assumed to be a rest-ing position, but when they were roused, they literally inflated and doubled their size and girth. Their muscular, meaty legs were long and spastic. I was staring at a full-fledged enormous Jurassic-era taran-tula-like creature in my bedroom. Enor-mous! It ran and scurried; I sprayed at it again, and it hid behind my nightstand.

I was beside myself. I was alone. I had a roommate, but Tracy, who for some reason was not afraid of Jurassic-era spi-ders, was on vacation in Zimbabwe for the week. I ran into the kitchen and just stood there with my mouth open. For as long as I could remember, I had been arachnopho-bic. I just never knew, growing up in Roch-ester, New York, and having lived in New York City, where spiders are not a thing at all, how tiny and insignificant those little yellow house spiders from my childhood were in comparison to these creatures.

I was actually in shock. I was out of my league. I had no idea what to do. I was all alone in this bug-infested house in this country where I didn't fully speak the lan-guage. Creatures like this one didn't just

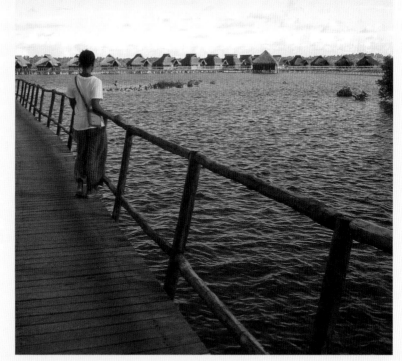

View of Flamingo Bay, Inhambane, Mozambique.

Below: Flamingo Bay, Inhambane, Mozambique.

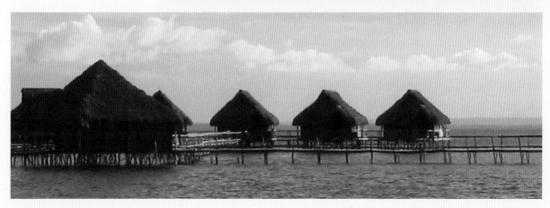

pass by—they entered and took over a space. It was so big and so fast. Baygonne just wasn't going to work. It was like trying to kill a pet cat with RAID. I paced the floor in the kitchen. I thought about sleeping outside, about walking back to the school and begging one of the students to let me sleep in their dormitory. I thought about giving up and catching a flight back home to New York, where I'd have a carefully controlled, spider-free environment.

As I was going through my options, the spider—as a way of giving me the finger, I'm sure—began to crawl along my door-frame, peering out at me. It was soooooo big. I couldn't believe what I was dealing with. Then I heard a television somewhere in the distance. I backed out of the house and onto my porch and remembered the lights were on next door. I sprinted to the next yard to see whether I could find my neighbor Belleview, but of course when

I was looking for him, I couldn't find him (and when I didn't want him around he was everywhere). Belleview was 13 and obsessed with America and the Cadbury chocolate bars and Maria tea biscuits in our cupboard that his mother wouldn't allow him to have. Belleview and his family were away, visiting his sister in one of the northern provinces. I did find two servants who worked for the family, though, and, in my broken Portuguese, I explained that I needed help because there was a large spider in my room that needed to be taken out. One of the men got up grudgingly from the football game he was watching on the television and followed me back into my house. I handed him a broom from my kitchen, and he entered my bedroom.

I waited in the kitchen, listening for news as he rummaged around. He stepped back out into the kitchen, shrugged his shoulders, and said he couldn't find it. This man was my only savior; I needed him to find that spider so I could sleep at night. After summoning up my courage, I entered the room with him, but I couldn't see it either. How could I not see a small dog in a sparsely furnished room? Then the man, a Mozambican who would in theory be used to these endemic creatures, actually screamed. You know it's bad when a local person who is used to all sorts of creepy crawly disgusting creatures screams in shock. This thing was sooooo big!

The spider jumped from underneath my bedframe and backed into a corner. It thrashed and danced. I swear I heard it hiss at the man before I ran out of the room, leaving him to fight the battle with the broom. The tussle lasted a good five minutes before the man emerged sheepishly.

"Is it dead?" I asked.

"No," he said reluctantly.

"Where is it?" I said.

"I don't know!" he stammered.

How could he not know? What was going on? Who was this super spider?

My neighbor's housekeeper was such a sweet man; he could tell I was distressed, so he was trying to be nice. As a concession, he brought me in the room, and we checked every corner and crevice; just like that, the spider was nowhere to be seen. At last, I gave in. Under his protective gaze, I grabbed my mosquito net tent and evacuated the room. I would never be able to look at my room in the same way. I didn't trust that the spider was gone. I knew it was in there hiding, waiting to catch me alone and defenseless.

I thanked the man profusely, watching as he eagerly scurried into the darkness to finish watching the match with his buddy. Feeling very alone, I set up camp in the walk-in pantry turned spare bedroom. It was a small, windowless room with a cot for the visitors we sometimes would receive.

I didn't sleep at all. I had visions of the giant beast crawling into the space from beneath the door and attacking me. I was so wound up, I shook the entire night. Every thought was of the spider. Every sound was the spider. Every stray hair that brushed against my face or hand was the spider.

The next morning at 5:00 a.m. my alarm went off because I supervised an agriculture project and was responsible for presenting a weekly lecture to the students about composting techniques. Slowly I unzipped the mesh tent that I had set on my bed. Head throbbing, legs shaky, I crawled out of my mosquito netting and made my way toward my room.

I froze; the events were too raw. I couldn't convince my feet to bring me inside. I took the tablecloth off the table, wrapped it around myself, grabbed my lecture and my bag, and took off.

On campus, I was met with stares.

"Teacher Soj-ah." Gil, one of the other professors, looked at me with thorough confusion. "Everything okay?"

"No."

"What happened?" Gil stepped toward me gingerly.

"I didn't sleep."

"Why not?" Gil's response was matter of fact.

"A spider, the size of . . ." I used my hands to show how large the beast was.

Gil's face broke into a grin.

I could feel my face getting hot.

"I was alone in the house. The spider was the size of my head. It was so fast."

Gil laughed.

"And it was hairy."

Gil laughed harder.

"Stop!"

"It's just a huntsman. They're harmless."

"You call that harmless?"

"They're big, but they come out when it's about to rain or after the rain because they live in the ground."

"You don't understand," I cut him off.

"It's a part of life, So-jah."

"Not my life. We don't have anything like that in New York. I was terrified. I didn't sleep. I feel dizzy and short of breath when I think about it. And I have to go back there, back into that house after work again tonight."

"I know how to help you sleep."

"How?"

"During siesta, I'll take you to see the curandeiro."

"The what?"

"That's our word for 'healer.'"

"Healer?"

"Yah, man. Remember when I hurt my ankle last month? I didn't go to the hospital. I just saw the healer; he gave me herbs, and I got better fast. Now I can play football again."

"But how will a curandeiro help me?"

"He'll mix you a bark tea. Help you sleep. Help you relax. You'll feel better."

"I don't know."

"Trust me, it will help. My mum goes because of her nerves, and it helps. She's a lot better."

I had nothing to lose. I was already running around with a throbbing headache, uncombed hair, and bloodshot eyes while wearing a tablecloth as a dress. So during our lunch break (or siesta, as they called it), we met in the teacher's office; my hair was sticking up everywhere from the makeshift bun I was forced to bind with two pencils since my one remaining elastic broke.

"Ready, So-jah?" Gil grinned.

I shrugged.

Gil rambled as we walked in the hot, humid sun three miles to the central market. Beyond the vendor stalls toward the food stalls and then down a narrow alleyway I'd never seen, I followed him, trying my best to follow his conversation about the football match from the previous night. There were several rooms without doors. We ducked into one such room as Gil gave a whistle, I assumed to announce our arrival. I don't know what I was expecting. Perhaps someone who looked similar to the tarot reader I'd once visited in New Orleans, an ancient mythical being with the power to see into my soul and create by hand an herbal concoction perfectly and astrologically aligned to suit my unique needs.

Instead, I was standing before a tall, handsome man wearing stylish glasses, tailored pants, and a fitted shirt. Busy with his phone, he couldn't have been more than 25. I looked at Gil, who said something to him in a language I couldn't understand. They both chuckled, and at last the man looked up from his phone as they engaged in an elaborate handshake.

"My friend Carlos. He's minding the shop for his father," Gil explained in slow Portuguese before turning back to his friend.

Again, they spoke in the language I couldn't identify—one of the many tribal languages that I was not privy to. A crate was overturned, and I was invited to sit as they continued their conversation. I

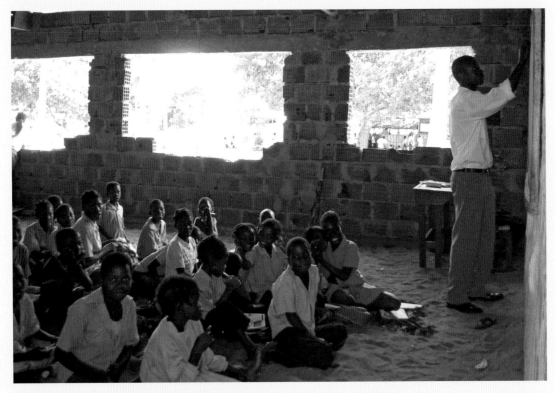

Conducting observations of student teachers in Inhambane, Mozambique.

Sunset, Tofo Beach, Inhambane, Mozambique.

Below: Huntsman spider.

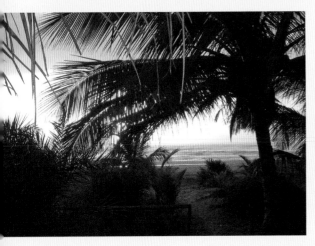

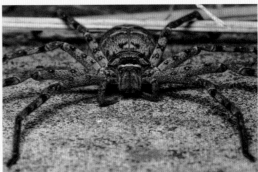

Mark Weich / 500px via Getty Images.

looked around the shop. It was indistinct, a bare three-walled room with crates and ledges that held bottles of liquids and bunches of herbs I couldn't identify. Herbs, barks, and flowers were crammed into old Coke and Fanta bottles. The ground was scattered with hay. The light in the shop was dim. I felt my eyes sag and my chin drop as I began to nod off to the sound of their indecipherable conversation.

"So-jah. So-jah." I snapped my head up to find Gil standing over me.

His friend, still occupied by his phone, didn't so much as look in my direction.

"Here, So-jah." He placed a small jar of amber liquid in my hand. The glass container looked like a baby food jar with the label incompletely peeled off. It wasn't marked or labeled in any way. It simply contained sediment-rich brown, murky liquid.

"So . . .?"

"Ansellia africana bark." Gil nodded toward the jar. "You have to drink it. It will help relax you."

I looked at the dusty jar in my hands, and a list of warnings ran through my mind: Don't drink tap water, don't eat out, peel your own fruit—and I'm sure somewhere on that long list of don'ts for Westerners in Mozambique lay the warning: Don't drink unidentifiable tonics made by medicine men.

"I don't know." I felt bad. He had gone through so much trouble, and I didn't want to be rude. I also didn't want to die.

"So-jah, I already bought it for you. You'll take it home and give it a try. It will work. You will sleep so well. The Ansellia africana bark is used to ward off bad dreams, and it will keep you relaxed."

"But I don't know what it is."

"It's bark."

"I don't want to drink it, though. I might get sick."

"No, So-jah, the bark will make you well."

"Yes, but I'm worried that I won't be able to tolerate it."

Gil paused, his brows furrowed. "Aaaah, yes. No problem."

He turned and consulted with Carlos. Again, left to myself, and not able to understand their conversation, I began to drift off. I don't know how long I was out. I woke to Gil's voice calling my name and the same jar, now filled with a dark resinous paste.

"It's soap," Gil announced proudly. "Use it every day, and you will be able to sleep."

"Soap?"

"Yes. Medicine soap. Use it at night before you sleep."

Realizing I didn't have the energy to protest, I said okay. I thanked Carlos for his time and efforts. We said good-bye and made our way back to campus.

When we finally arrived, sweaty and dusty from the road, I set the concoction on my desk and made my way into the cafeteria for lunch.

That night, when I returned home around 6:30 p.m., it was completely light out. The housekeeper had already left, foiling my plan of having some support so that I could get back into my room to retrieve much-needed supplies. I needed to get into my room. My shower caddy and clothes were in there. I couldn't walk around all week, wrapped in a tablecloth, until Tracy returned.

It took me a good 15 minutes to convince my legs to walk to the door and my hands to turn the doorknob so I could enter the room. Tiptoeing, while looking wildly about, I gathered items one by one and dashed into the living room to set them on the sofa before returning for another pile. I didn't see the spider, but I didn't feel safe either.

Because I am a germaphobe, the thought of using the bark tonic medicine soap—given the questionably sanitized, reused bottle and all—made me almost as nervous as the spider did, but the promise of sleep did spark my curiosity. I made my way into the thatched-roof shower hut. I set my things on the bench and then made my way to the communal well to collect a bucket of water. Cupping water in my hands, I splashed myself until damp. I opened the jar. A musty, earth aroma met my nostrils. I dipped my fingers into the paste; it was gritty. I took a deep breath and did what I was told. I rubbed the soap on my wet skin. It didn't lather and formed more of a mask. Using a plastic cup, I rinsed the soap off of my skin. It was stubborn and left slimy streaks, and I had run out of my bucket of water. Wrapping myself in a piece of fabric, I walked back out to the well, refilled my bucket with water, and tried again. This time, I took out my bottle of Dr. Bronner's peppermint castile soap and lathered my skin to get rid of the medicine soap residue. I rinsed again, toweled off, and got dressed. It was so nice to be clean.

I slept in the office that night and stayed up late conducting research on barks since I had access to an internet connection at school but not at my house. It turned out that bark, the outermost layer of a tree, held a host of medical benefits that traditional healers in Mozambique had been relying upon for generations. Tree bark was used to treat a variety of ailments, including inflammation, arthritis, cancer, high blood pressure, insomnia, nerves, and back pain. Bark strips were removed from the desired tree to be used immediately or dried and saved for later, and the bark would most usually be turned into teas, poultices, salves, and tinctures. Not all bark is the same; there's inner bark and outer bark. When it comes to medicine making, you want to access the inner bark, which is softer and sap filled—the layer just beyond the rougher outer bark exterior. For the purposes of this book, I'm focusing on salves and tinctures since they can be incorporated easily into body care formulations, like I imagine Carlos did with the medicine soap.

But first, I'll distinguish between the two. A salve is an ointment used to treat skin irritations, and a tincture is a concentrated liquid formulation containing the healing properties extracted from the desired bark. There were several popular medicinal barks used in Mozambique, including the Ansellia africana that I had received. In fact, one troubling side effect of the rapid development undertaking the country was the fact that deforestation was a huge factor, not only in environmental troubles but also in a loss of trees used in villages for the healing properties of their barks. In many rural villages, medicine men and women were the primary source of medical treatment, and these traditional healers relied on the forests to treat their patients.

Generally, when making a bark salve, you place the bark in a pot, cover the bark with an oil like olive oil, and simmer for 20 minutes with the lid on. Strain the bark out of the oil and then melt beeswax into the concoction (3 tablespoons of beeswax to 1 cup of olive oil), stirring before allowing it to cool and harden.

The general rule for tinctures is to chop the bark into small pieces and place inside a glass container. Cover bark with 100 proof vodka for 8 days, shaking each day. After 8 days, strain, and your tincture is ready for use.

REMOVING INNER BARK

Trees are living beings. When working with trees, take care and practice "non-harm." Harvesting bark can be traumatic for trees. Be gentle, give thanks, and take only what you need. The method I use is to take a sharp knife and carve a piece of bark roughly the size of a 4-inch by 6-inch rectangle.

Using the tip of my knife, I gently pry off the bark, a few layers deep. When the bark is removed from the tree, it's as if the tree has scraped its knee. The tree now has an open wound. Almost immediately you'll see sticky sap begin to form at the site of the wound. This is the tree's attempt to heal itself. Don't forget to thank your tree for allowing you to remove some of its bark—its essence.

When you're ready to prepare your bark, wash your hands and carefully peel the outer bark away. The softer, fragrant, and oftentimes moist bark beneath is what you're after; that's the inner bark.

Check in on your tree for a few weeks following the bark extraction. The open wound can leave the tree susceptible

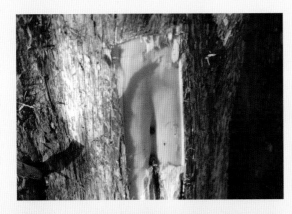

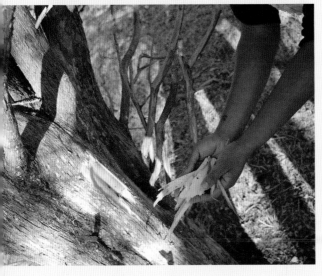

Carving a rectangular patch in a cedar tree to harvest bark.

Below: Slicing cedar bark.

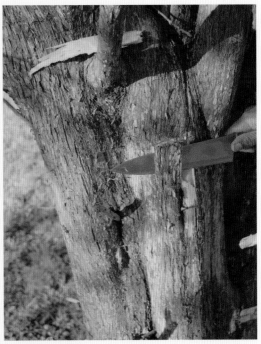

At left: Harvesting cedar bark with a knife.

to mites and infections just as an open wound, without proper care, can do for us. Tea tree essential oil, applied an inch or so around the periphery of the wound, will help keep mites and pests away from the wound while the tree heals.

When you're ready to extract more bark, spread it out—go to a different tree. If you absolutely must return to the same tree, make your next incision in a different place and repeat the process.

Both salves and tinctures can be incorporated into body care products to enhance the healing properties. There are so many different ways to use bark salves and tinctures in skin and hair formulations. I'll outline some of my favorite recipes in the following pages.

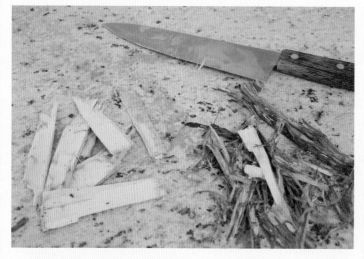

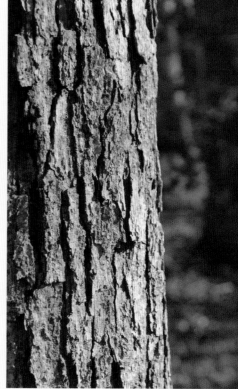

Inner bark versus outer bark.

At right: Oak tree, outer bark, Southern Maryland.

PINE SALVE

Moisturizing, anti-inflammatory, and antiseptic, this powerful healing salve can be used directly as a spot treatment to treat acne, bruising, and inflammation, or it can be added to one of the body butter recipes in this book to boost healing properties.

WHAT YOU'LL NEED:

- ¼ cup pine resin (this can be accessed by carving a slice in the tree and waiting a few days for the sap to form near the slice)
- ½ cup calendula oil
- 1½ tablespoons finely grated beeswax

WHAT TO DO:

1. Pry the resin off the pine bark using a spoon. Try to get pieces of resin that are sticky to touch from the sap.
2. Cover the ¼ cup of resin with calendula oil in a saucepan. Heat over low heat until the resin and oil melt together.
3. Strain the pine resin and calendula oil and add the beeswax to melt.

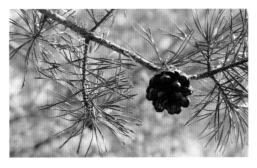

Southern Maryland shortleaf pine.

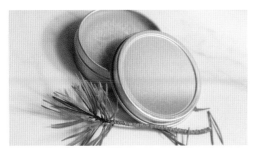

Pine Salve.

Yield:
One 8-ounce jar of salve

Preparation time:
30 minutes

Indications:
This soothing salve with antispasmodic, antiseptic, and antimicrobial properties promotes the repair of skin tissue.

Usage:
This concoction can be used alone as a salve to increase circulation, spot treat skin irritations, and even remove splinters. Apply directly to skin using clean fingertips.

It can also be added to any of the body butter recipes at a ratio of about 1 teaspoon to 4 ounces. To add a salve to body butter, mix the salve directly into the shea butter or coconut oil as it's melting, and then proceed as directed in the recipe. The salve will increase the healing properties of the body butter.

This salve recipe can also be added to any of the lotion recipes in this book to enhance their healing properties. To add to lotion, combine the salve mixture before it cools to the oil base of the lotion before it cools. Add about 1 teaspoon per 4 ounces.

Storage:
Store in a cool, dry place for up to a year. Wash hands before dipping your fingers into the salve to preserve the salve's integrity.

BIRCH BARK SALVE

Anti-inflammatory, this salve soothes skin rashes such as those caused by eczema and psoriasis. It can be used alone as a spot treatment or combined with one of the body butter recipes from this book to concentrate the healing properties.

WHAT YOU'LL NEED:

- ½ cup birch bark (inner bark, not the white outer bark)
- ½ cup extra virgin olive oil
- 1½ tablespoons beeswax
- ⅛ teaspoon turmeric

WHAT TO DO:

1. Gather birch bark (the layer beneath the white exterior).
2. Place the bark in a saucepan and cover with extra virgin olive oil.
3. Simmer on low 1 to 5 hours, until the oil is the color of the bark.
4. Strain the oil and melt the beeswax into the mixture.
5. Blend.
6. Add turmeric.
7. Blend again.

Yield:
One 8-ounce jar

Preparation time:
30 minutes

Indications:
This salve has calming, anti-inflammatory, antibacterial, antiseptic, and clarifying properties.

Usage:
Apply directly to irritated skin using a clean fingertip, or blend into body butter, skin oil, and toner recipes at about 1 teaspoon per 4 ounces. Add the salve to the melting shea butter or coconut oil step in the recipe.

Storage:
Store in a cool, dry place for up to a year. Make sure your fingers are clean when you dip them into the salve to preserve the integrity of the formula.

CEDAR BARK TINCTURE

Woodsy, grounding, aromatic, and a natural insect repellant, this tincture can be combined by the dropperful into body oil, body butter, and toner recipes from this book.

WHAT YOU'LL NEED:

- ¼ cup chopped cedar bark (inner bark)
- ⅓ to ½ cup 100 proof vodka
- 1 teaspoon vegetable glycerin

WHAT TO DO:

1. Place chopped bark into a jar and cover the bark completely with the vodka.
2. Leave bark to sit in a dimly lit, cool, dry place for 30 days.
3. Shake the contents of the jar every day.
4. After 30 days, strain the liquid and add the glycerin.

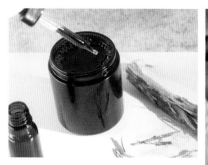

Creating a tincture from cedar bark.

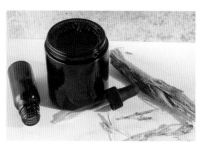

Cedar Bark Tincture.

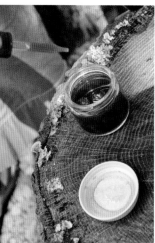

Concocting a medicinal bark tincture in the woods.

Yield:
One 4-ounce spray bottle

Preparation time:
10 minutes (30-day wait time)

Indications:
This natural insect repellant works as an anti-inflammatory, reduces itchiness, and moisturizes skin.

Usage:
This tincture can be added to any of the toner, body butter, or body oil recipes at a ratio of 1 dropperful per 4 ounces. If adding to body butter, combine while the mixture is at its coolest point while still in a liquid form. This tincture can be applied directly to the skin using a cotton ball or as a cologne. The scent doubles as an insect repellant.

Storage:
Store in a cool, dry place. The 100 proof vodka will preserve the integrity of this tincture for 3 to 5 years at least.

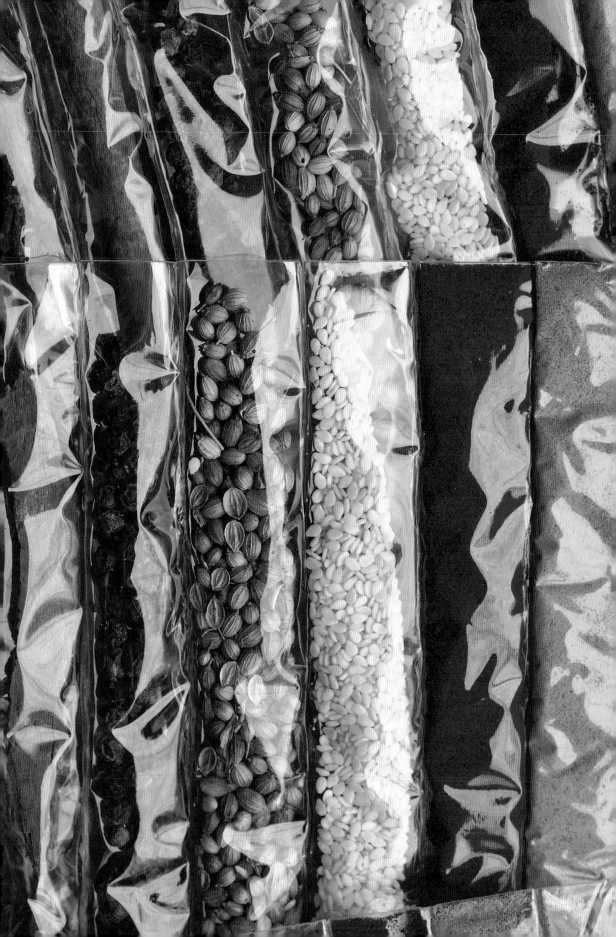

STORING YOUR PRODUCTS

All of the recipes in this book are 100% natural and free of synthetic additives and preservatives. This being said, there are some things to consider when it comes to storage.

GENERAL GUIDELINES

- Store products in a cool, dry environment. Cool environments help slow the separation process of ingredients in your natural formulations.
- Avoid direct sunlight and hot humid bathrooms, as the potency of your product may be compromised. Heat and humidity also open the door to bacterial growth.
- Dark glass bottles will help preserve the integrity of your products. I recommend amber or cobalt bottles, as they do an excellent job of filtering out sunlight.

- I recommend using glass bottles over plastic. Plastic bottles can leach toxins. If plastic is preferred, I recommend finding BPA-free HDPE plastic containers, as they are generally considered the least damaging.
- Products with dairy (milk and yogurt mainly) must be refrigerated and have a six-week shelf life.
- Refrigeration for all products, whether or not they contain dairy, is a good idea during the summer months if you live in a very warm environment.

A NOTE ABOUT NATURAL PRESERVATIVES

In a perfect world, one drop of tea tree essential oil would be enough to protect your handmade products from bacterial contamination, but it's not that simple. Oftentimes products that have antimicrobial and antioxidant properties (such as tea tree essential oil) are termed "natural preservatives." While these products can help maintain the integrity of your natural products, they are not powerful enough to provide full spectrum protection against bacteria, fungi, and mold.

The good news is that not all products will require additional preservatives. As a general rule, products without water will not need preservatives since bacteria needs water to grow. So, if your product is any combination of carrier oil, essential oil, butter, and/or wax, you don't need to worry about a preservative.

When you're working with fats (carrier oils and butters), however, you do want to add an antioxidant to your formulation, as fats can become rancid without antioxidants. I suggest using vitamin E, which works wonderfully in bath and beauty formulations to preserve the good qualities of oil blends. Vitamin E is an antioxidant and will not prevent or kill bacteria growth if your blend contains water.

If your blend contains water, you have a few options. My favorite option is refrigeration. Refrigerating your product will offer protection from bacterial growth. Another option is to use a preservative to extend the shelf life. There are a few preservatives that are considered safe to use in natural products. Generally speaking, following European Union (EU) cosmetic legislation is a good way to go since Europe has a highly regulated cosmetic industry. Some of the EU-approved preservatives include silver citrate (water-soluble antimicrobial preservative), citric acid (preservative against mold and bacteria), and MEA-benzoate (preservative salts).

SENSITIVE SKIN CONSIDERATIONS

Everyone is different, and a skin reaction to natural ingredients is always possible depending on your unique internal makeup. As with food products, if you have a sensitivity to nuts, avoid nut oils. It's also a good idea to consult your doctor if you have inflammatory skin disorders such as eczema, psoriasis, or rosacea.

If you're pregnant, nursing, or creating a product for a baby or small child, you'll want to do your essential oil research, as some essential oils are considered harmful to babies, small children, and pregnant and nursing mothers.

No matter what your condition, when trying something new, it's always a good idea to conduct a skin patch test to see how your body reacts to a particular ingredient or set of ingredients.

HOW TO CONDUCT A SKIN PATCH TEST

1. Wash and completely dry a patch of skin on the upper part of your inner arm (near the crook of your elbow).
2. Apply a pea sized amount of the product you're testing.
3. Cover with a Band-Aid and leave for 24 hours. Try not to get the area wet.
4. After 24 hours, remove your bandage and check for signs of irritation like redness, burning, itching, rashes, or blistering.
5. If irritation occurs, remove the bandage and wash the area with soap and water.

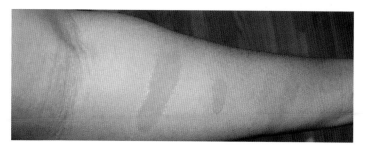

Apply a small dab of product to your inner arm to test for allergic reactions.

IN CLOSING

I hope this book has been both enjoyable to read and informative. For your ease, I have added a list of websites that will direct you to some of my favorite resources for purchasing the products, materials, and tools I use to make my bath and beauty products. Please note that I am not sponsored by any of these companies and am making recommendations based only on my preferences.

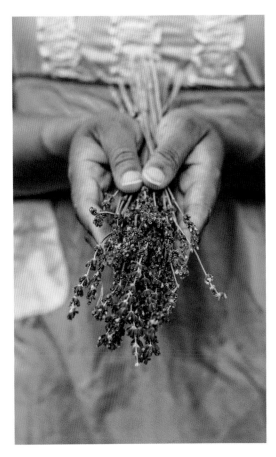

Remember, your health is in your hands. You are what you put on your skin, so it's crucial to nourish yourself not only from the inside out but also from the outside in.

I wish you continued health and happiness.

Blessings,
Sojourner

Lavender bouquet.

RESOURCES

MOUNTAIN ROSE HERBS

Organic non-GMO spices, herbs, body butters, waxes, salts, carrier oils, clays, and containers. See www.mountainroseherbs.com.

JADE BLOOM ESSENTIAL OILS

High-quality essential oils, carrier oils, and hydrosols. See www.jadebloom.com.

FLORACOPEIA ESSENTIAL OILS

Organic and wildcrafted essential oils and flower essences. See www.floracopeia.com.

SKS BOTTLE AND PACKAGING

Glass bottles and jars, tins, and capsules for easy storage. See www.sks-bottle.com.

BULK APOTHECARY

Body butters, oils, waxes, and containers. See www.bulkapothecary.com.

DR. BRONNER

A variety of castile-based soaps for use in shampoo and body wash recipes. See www.drbronner.com.

LINDERA FARMS

Fine and rare vinegars, locally and sustainably sourced in Virginia. See www.linderafarms.com.

INDEX

castile soap base: body wash, 131; moisturizing shampoo, 127

castor oil: black, 53–55, 64, 138; conditioner, 128; hair cream, 18; plant, 59f; red clay hair mask, 90; uses of, 59

cedar bark tincture, 165

cedarwood essential oil, 102; beard cream, 26; mood-boosting body mist, 75; perfume spray, 79

cellulite, essential oils for, 107, 108, 109

Celtic sea salt, facial cleanser, 36

chai bath salts, 50

chamomile essential oil, 102

chamomile flower, herbal bath, 49

charcoal masks, 88–89

cherry blossom vinegar, 147; toner, 149

Chinese traditional medicine, 105, 116, 137

cinnamic acid, 12

cinnamon, 44, 44f; body scrub, 37; golden milk sugar scrub, 46

cinnamon (bark) essential oil, 103; bath salts, 50; shea butter deodorant, 14

circulation, essential oils for, 106, 107, 108, 111, 113, 115, 119

citric acid, 168; bath bombs, 48

citronella essential oil, 103

clary sage essential oil, 104

clay, 83–97; types of, 87; uses of, 87

cleanser: bentonite clay, 93; coconut oil/green clay, 97

Cleopatra, 43–44, 137

clove, bath salts, 50

clove essential oil, 104; bath salts, 50; mouthwash, 129; perfume spray, 79; toothpaste, 91

cocoa powder: facial powder, 96; lip gloss, 126

coconut, 32f

coconut cream, golden milk sugar scrub, 46

coconut milk, moisturizing shampoo, 127

coconut oil, 28–38; body butter, 22–23; body lotion, 33–34, 142; body scrub, 37, 46; conditioner, 128; cooling mask, 92; deodorant, 130; face mask, 38; facial cleanser, 36, 93, 97; indications for, 32; moisturizing shampoo, 127; red clay hair mask, 90; salt scrub, 45; toothpaste, 35, 91; uses of, 58

coffee body scrub, 37

cold-pressed oils, 57, 100–101

colds, essential oils for, 111–12, 114, 115

cold sores, Melissa essential oil for, 111

conditioner, 128

conditioning mask, 140

congestion, essential oils for, 105, 106, 114, 117

containers, 2, 2f, 167; resources for, 171

cooling products: face mist, 81; green clay mask, 92

copaiba essential oil, 104

cornstarch: bath bombs, 48; deodorant powder, 94; facial powder, 96

Costa Rica, 132–36, 133f–34f, 136f

coughs, essential oils for, 110, 111, 114, 119

cucumber, calming face mist, 73

curandeiro, 157–59

curly hair: daily conditioner for, 128; hair gel for, 19; moisturizing cream for, 18; moisturizing shampoo for, 127; red clay hair mask, 90

cuticle softener, shea butter, 21

cypress essential oil, 105

dandruff: aloe vera for, 137; black castor oil for, 54; essential oils for, 113, 115, 118; scalp-rejuvenating serum, 138; shea butter for, 13

deodorant: essential oil blend, 130;

muscle soreness, essential oils for, 105, 106, 108, 109, 110, 113–14, 115, 117, 119, 120

myrrh essential oil, 111; body oil, 65; conditioner, 128; moisturizer, 24; stretch mark cream, 20

myrrh resin, bath bombs, 48

Native Americans, and aloe vera, 137

natural preservatives, 168

nausea, essential oils for, 106, 113, 114

neem oil: hair-growth oil, 64; uses of, 59

New York City, 98–100, 99*f*–100*f*

nutmeg essential oil, perfume spray, 79

oil herbal infusions, 72

oils: carrier, 51–65; coconut, 28–38; essential, 98–131

oleic acid, 12, 59

olive oil: birch bark salve, 164; body butter, 23; body wash, 131; conditioner, 128; lip gloss, 126; lotion bars, 15; shaving cream, 16; uses of, 58

orange peel: bath salts, 50; facial cleanser, 36; facial scrub, 47

oregano, facial scrub, 47

oregano essential oil, 112

pain: essential oils for, 103, 104, 106, 109, 110, 111–12, 117, 119, 120, 121; hemp seed oil for, 60

palmitic acid, 12

palmitoleic acid, 58

palo santo essential oil, 112

pantry, 3–4

parabens, 2

parasites: essential oils for, 112, 119; neem oil for, 59

parsley seed essential oil, 113

patchouli essential oil, 113; lip balm, 125; perfume spray, 77

patch testing, 169

peppermint, *xf*

peppermint essential oil, 99, 113; body wash, 131; hair cream, 18; hand sanitizer, 124; moisturizing shampoo, 127; mouthwash, 123; scalp-rejuvenating serum, 138; toothpaste, 35, 91

perfume sprays: citrus/herb, 80; floral, 78; spicy, 79; woodsy/earthy, 77

periodontitis, clary sage essential oil for, 104

phthalates, 2

pine needle essential oil, 114

pine resin salve, 163

plant barks, 151–65, 161*f*–62*f*; removing, 161–62; uses of, 160

plum vinegar, 147

Portugal, 66–71, 67*f*–70*f*

powders: deodorant, 94; facial, oil-absorbing, 96

preservatives, 2; natural, 168

prostatitis, pine needle essential oil for, 114

psoriasis, 169; birch bark salve for, 164; coconut oil for, 32; essential oils for, 113, 114

purity: of carrier oils, 57; of coconut oil, 32; of essential oils, 100

rashes: birch bark salve for, 164; shea butter for, 13. *See also* eczema; psoriasis

raspberry vinegar toner, 148

red clay, 87; hair mask, 90

refined oils, 57

relaxing body mist, 76

rice vinegar toner, 150

ricinoleic acid, 54, 59

Rilke, Rainer Maria, 1

ringworm, pine needle essential oil for, 114

rosacea, 169; green clay face mask for, 95

sunscreen: essential oils for, 107, 115; shea butter as, 10–11, 13, 25

Swaziland, 83–84, 84*f*–86*f*

sweet almond oil: bath salts, 50; beard cream, 26; hair gel, 19; scar-reducing oil, 63; uses of, 58

sweet orange essential oil, 118

Taino medicine, 53

tamanu oil: anti-aging facial serum, 61; moisturizer, 24; sunscreen, 25; uses of, 60

tangerine essential oil, 118

tea, in toners: green, 148; mint, 150

tea tree essential oil, 99, 118; deodorant, 130; facial cleanser, 97; hand sanitizer, 124; masks, 88–89; moisturizing shampoo, 127; mouthwash, 123, 129; scalp-rejuvenating serum, 138; toothpaste, 91; for tree bark removal, 162

termites, sweet orange essential oil for, 118

Thailand, 28–31, 29*f*–31*f*

thyme, 44

thyme essential oil, 119; deodorant, 130; herbal bath, 49; perfume spray, 80

Tibetan traditional medicine, 116

tinctures: cedar bark, 165; definition of, 160–61

toners: cherry blossom vinegar, 149; floral, 82; raspberry vinegar, 148; rice vinegar, 150; rose, 122; skin-brightening mist, 74

tonsillitis, rosemary essential oil for, 115

toothache: clove mouthwash for, 129; essential oils for, 106, 112

toothpaste: coconut oil, 35; white kaolin clay, 91

traditional medicine, xv; Australian, 118; Ayurveda, xii–xiii, xiv, 32, 44, 53, 116; Chinese, 105, 116, 137; Jamaican, 53; Mozambican, 157–59; Thai, 30; Tibetan, 116

translucent facial powder, 96

travel, xiv–xv

tree barks, 151–65, 161*f*–62*f*; removing, 161–62; uses of, 160

triclosan, 2

turmeric, 42*f*, 44, 44*f*; anti-aging cream, 27; bath salts, 50; birch bark salve, 164; face mask, 95; facial powder, 96; sugar scrub, 46

turmeric essential oil, 119

unrefined oils, 57

vanilla, 44*f*; body scrub, 37; perfume spray, 79

varicose veins, essential oils for, 105, 107, 108, 113, 115, 116

vetiver essential oil, 120; beard cream, 26; mood-boosting body mist, 75; perfume spray, 77

vinegars, 144–50; face masks, 38, 89; facial toner, 148–50; hair mask, 90; resources for, 171; uses of, 147

viral infections: castor oil for, 59; essential oils for, 102, 103, 105, 108, 110, 112, 113–15, 118–19, 120

virgin oil, 57

vitamin E oil, 168; body butter, 22–23; body lotion, 33–34, 142; body scrub, 17, 37; body wash, 131; conditioner, 128; deodorant, 14; facial cleanser, 97; lip balm, 125; lip gloss, 126; moisturizer, 24; shampoo, 127; shaving cream, 16; stretch mark cream, 20

wavy hair. *See* curly hair

whipped body butter, shea butter, 22

whipped body lotion: aloe vera, 142; coconut/aloe, 33; for mature skin, 34

white clay, 87; toothpaste, 91

white sage essential oil, 120

white thyme essential oil, deodorant, 130

wintergreen essential oil, 121

witch hazel: bath bombs, 48; face mists, 74, 81; facial toners, 82, 122, 150

worms, essential oils for, 119

wounds: coconut oil for, 32; essential oils for, 102, 107, 108, 110, 113, 115, 116, 118–19, 120; tamanu oil for, 60

wrinkles. *See* aging, signs of

xylitol, toothpaste, 91

ylang ylang essential oil, 121; body mist, 75; body scrub, 17; conditioner, 128; deodorant, 130; facial serum, 62; facial toner, 82; perfume spray, 78

yoga, xii

yogurt masks, 88, 92, 95

Zanzibar, 39–43, 41*f*–42*f*, 44*f*

ABOUT THE AUTHOR

Sojourner Walker Williams is an Ayurvedic practitioner, yoga instructor, and energy healer based in New York City and Southern Maryland, depending on the day. An enthusiast of travel and DIY body care products, she has compiled her acquired knowledge into this engaging and informative resource guide. *Natural Beauty from the Outside In* is her first book.

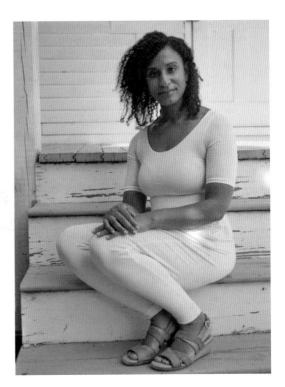